Healthy Aging

....

About the Authors

JOSEPH BONNER spent his undergraduate years at the
University of Colorado and was a member of the National
Ski Patrol at Vail. He received his doctoral degree in
molecular biology from the University of Southern
California, where he also worked in the Andrus
Gerontology Center. He then studied at California
Institute of Technology on a postdoctoral fellowship
awarded by the National Institutes of Health. His
research interests ranged from the biology of development
(specifically, cleft palate) to intercellular communication
in the immune system. His teaching credits include the
University of Southern California, Cal Tech, University of
California, Los Angeles, School of Dentistry, and
University of California, Los Angeles, Extension, where
in 1981, he created the Biology of Aging course from
which this book was drawn. His work has been widely
published in scientific journals.

WILLIAM HARRIS received his B.A. in English
literature from The University of the South at Sewanee.
He studied at the *Sorbonne* and the *Institut des Sciences
Politiques* in Paris. He spent two years in Naples, Italy
before becoming a newspaper reporter and editor in
Southern California where he has remained, making
Venice Beach his home. He has been a writer of theater
reviews, speeches, and continuing education courses for
the Veterans Administration where he works as a
disability evaluator. Working on this book, he says,
added to his life an interest in reading current science
and medicine research reports. It also led him to stop
smoking and to make physical exercise a routine. Every
morning he and his two dogs run for an hour and then he
bicycles a bit before breakfast.

Men do not care how nobly they live,
but only how long.

Seneca

HEALTHY AGING

New Directions in Health, Biology, and Medicine

....

Joseph Bonner, Ph.D.
and
William Harris

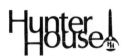

First U.S. edition published in 1988 by Hunter House Inc., Publishers

Hunter House Inc.
P.O. Box 847
Claremont, CA 91711.

Library of Congress Cataloging-in-Publication Data:

Bonner, Joseph J.
   Healthy aging: new directions in health,
biology and medicine

   Bibliography: p.
   Includes index.
   1. Aged—Health and hygiene. 2. Aging. I.
Harris, William, 1945– . II. Title.
RA777.6.B66   1988   613'.0438—dc19   88-9012
ISBN 089793-050-9
ISBN 089793-053-3 (pbk.)

Cover design and illustration by Teri Robertson
Illustrations by Daniel Nyiri
Copy editing by Jennifer D. Trzyna
Production manager: Paul J. Frindt
Set in 12 on 13 Bodoni by Coghill Book Typesetting, Richmond, Virginia

Manufactured in the United States of America

9 8 7 6 5 4 3   First edition

Contents

List of Figures

Preface

When Joe Bonner invited me to sit in on his "Biology of Aging" course at UCLA Extension, my reaction was not altogether cheerful. The big Four-O had become a reality for me and I somewhat gloomily expected his lectures to describe in livid, scientific terms all the detail of decay to come. How surprised I was, then, to find this youngish professor of molecular biology enthralling his classroom of enthusiastic middleaged people with vivid accounts of bodies and minds maintaining strength and vitality throughout a lifetime, largely due to good health habits of exercise and nutrition.

The class studied the changes which take place in our bodies between birth and death, and the focus was not on old age but on our ability to adjust to these changes at any stage of life. Most important, amid all the scientific evidence which Dr. Bonner presented was a sense of changing attitudes toward aging—some new directions for growing older.

The students attracted to his course included people in continuing education such as nurses, dental hygienists, physicians, psychologists, beauticians, an assortment of graduate students, and mostly, laymen who were interested (as I was) in the aging body after the age of, say, 30. The positive attitude toward growing older infected us all.

Making the transition from lecture to a book for the general reader became a project for Joe and me—a cheerful project, I must add, since his material was compelling. The challenge was to convey the findings of biological research to readers who want to learn about aging not only with grace, but also with good health.

Following the general format of the lectures, we broke the book into chapters dealing with the systems of the body such as the endocrine system, the cardiovascular system, and the central nervous system; we stressed the interactions of all the systems—our biological well-being or homeostasis, as biology calls it. The aging changes of one system affect all the others.

The endocrine system regulates our growth and reproduction but do hormones, the subject of Chapter Four, signal the onset of age? Are hormones the instigators of menopause or are they merely carrying out the orders of another source, the brain? Most hormone levels do not decrease as we age.

Drugs occupy such an exalted place in our culture that they have almost replaced religion—we rely on them to soothe the body and the soul. We felt they deserved a chapter. It is important to know that many of our physiological aging changes in the kidney, in the liver, and in the gastrointestinal tract heighten the effects of drugs, and we should adjust our dosages of them as we age.

Our bodies require a balanced diet and at no time is this more important than middle age and old age. Chapter Six shows that we need a certain amount of sodium, a certain amount of cholesterol-producing nutrients, and, yes, a certain amount of fat. The biological changes in our bodies illustrate why.

The cardiovascular system serves us quite well into advanced age, provided, of course, that we treat it with the respect it is due. A chapter explains why our cardiac output and our arterial pressure, if free from disease, can respond admirably, if a bit more slowly, to the stresses of changing age.

Alzheimer's disease and Parkinson's disease are not, by any means, common denominators of aging. Senility, discussed in Chapter Eleven, is neither inevitable nor untreatable and the experience that the brain stores away during our lives counts for far more than the few neurons we lose after six or seven decades.

A regular and vigorous program of exercise is most definitely a common denominator in the good health of all our bodily systems. Chapter Seven describes research showing why exercise is better for aging skin than creams and lotions;

science is proving that exercise benefits the brain, the heart, and the immune response at any age.

Foremost, we wanted readers who lack a background in molecular biology to share in the excitement of recent aging research, so we placed Chapters Two and Three on genetics and the theories of aging early on in the book. In addition, we have labelled certain passages as technical digressions—passages which readers may decide to peruse or not. They are intended to refrain from bogging readers down with scientific detail while providing keys to understanding changes of the body at the molecular level and keys to answering questions such as Why do we age? Do we have a biological clock ticking away the minutes and years, a DNA-directed development and demise? How do our cells know how many times to divide before they stop? Do we age because we are bombarded with environmental hazards such as ultraviolet radiation and diesel fumes? Why does genetics hold the potential for stretching our life expectancy to 90 years, or maybe 110?

We want to thank UCLA Extension for the opportunity to develop the material used in the course and in this book. We thank all the students whose helpful comments guided the manuscript; and thanks to my mother, Virginia Harris, for her patient and painstaking typing (which she, now in her 71st year of aging, calls "word-processing").

WH
Venice, Ca. 1988

For our parents

Chapter 1

Aging Hopefully

Lying about our age might be called a cultural hallmark of our society. When we turn 40 we feel better by saying we're 39. Long before that we hang onto 29 until we're 33, and later we want to maintain 35 for a good long while. Some of us are so good at it in our late forties and fifties that we actually forget our exact age. We have to subtract the year of our birth from the calendar year, just to be sure.

The master at the false-age fib, of course, was Jack Benny, who at least made us laugh at our fear of aging. Laughter decidedly eases the passage from our thirties to our forties; as a palliative, laughter is preferable to depression, anxiety, or alcohol. Unlike them, laughter doesn't harm our health—and healthy is definitely the way to age.

Forestalling the effects of aging has been a dream of mankind since history began. It is not so farfetched now as when Ponce de Leon looked for the legendary fountain of youth in Florida. Millions of us are still looking for it (albeit more scientifically) in Florida, Arizona, California, and other places. We make the same mistake Ponce de Leon made: There is no such thing as a fountain of youth. What we should look for instead is a fountain of health, and today, science is proving that the fountain of health exists. To look for the fountain of youth is to only set ourselves up for disastrous defeat. That fountain cannot be found, not even in our new growing knowledge of genetics. Genetics promises to free us from disease but it cannot stop aging. We grow old—there is no way around it. Mother Nature has planned it that way.

Besides, what we really want, what we're really looking and wishing for, is a long life of good health, not one of youth. Isn't maturity preferable to youth? And youth is not, by any means, synonymous with good health. Many unfortunate young people suffer and die from degenerative diseases. Although young, they are not healthy people.

Maturity brings large measures of peace and serenity that youth knows nothing about. Our goal should be maturity with good health. The fountain of health is a reachable goal. We can find it.

Not everyone in the world holds our Western abhorrence of growing old. Hidden away from the glare of contemporary publicity, there are several societies, each residing in a mountainous environment, who actually revere old age. Growing old to them is no disgrace. Western scientists of the aging process have visited such places as the town of Vilcabamba in the Ecuadorian Andes, communities in the mountains of the Russian Caucasus, and villages in the hilly Karakorum area of Kashmir, and they have discovered that the inhabitants, like us, are not above lying about their age. But there's a twist. Their lying is different from ours—they add years, and we take years away. Some people in those societies claim to be 120 years old, some claim to be 140, and some even claim 150.

Unfortunately, the proud centenarians can rarely prove they're as old as they claim. Their allegations of old age are mostly anecdotal. There is no scientific evidence to substantiate their longevity. The best a 140-year old can do is point to church records of his birth or ask a neighbor or witness who has known him for a hundred of his years for verification.

Now there is a long tradition in Russia and South America of falsifying birth records so as to escape military service. This was true under the Czars and other dictators and it's a problem today for the Soviets. There is also another fact to be remembered when listening to claims these people make about their longevity: Illiteracy is the norm for them and birth records are not as systematic as ours are in the West. Most of them cannot read their birth certificates even if they possess them. For the oldest among them, the knowledge of birth dates is passed from generation to generation by word of mouth. But whatever the truth about their age, the elderly and wise members of the societies receive the respect of the younger members, a major cultural difference between them and us. There, the elders are valued for their age and experience.

For both sets of fibbers, we Westerners seeking youth and the mountain folk of Kashmir seeking the respect of their young, science is replacing anecdote with fact. A new biological test tells the true story—laying bare a person's molecular essence by measuring something that is called "amino acid conversion." Rather like measuring the rings of growth in an old tree, when the test has been made on cell tissue of teeth from some of the people who allege 140 years, it has been found they really are about 90 years old. Still, 90 years is not bad. And generally they're healthy at 90. Our life expectancy in the United States is in the mid-seventies; we are fortunate indeed to reach 74 or 75 without a degenerative disease or two.

In our fascination with these healthy old people of mountain tribes, many scientific studies have been made to find out why they have such a long life expectancy. Certainly their medical care is backward compared to ours, but four aspects of their lives appear to help them age with so much ease. One, they remain physically active all their lives, rarely escaping to a rocking chair. They work in the fields with the younger members of their families or they tote provisions up steep hillsides daily. They don't stop their work at age 65; they don't "retire." And their daily work is not a "career" that begins in their twenties—a lifetime of work is your birthright when you're born in a village in the Andes. Your routine begins as soon as you can lift a bucket. It won't cease to be your routine for, chances are, a hundred years. A second reason for their longevity seems to be that they don't have much stress to deal with. They are not filled with anxiety about next year's pay raise. Life, for them (just as work) is routine. They know where the next meal is coming from— they will play a part, in fact, in providing it. Third, they eat differently from us. They don't take in as many calories as we do. They eat more carbohydrates than we do, but much less fat and protein.

Finally, as elders they are respected for their wisdom and their knowledge gained throughout their long lives. They are, in their own eyes and in everyone else's, important and valued members of their communities. We live in a vastly different world.

Changing Attitudes Toward Aging

For most of us in Western society aging is a reality of negativism. We usually try to put if off, and when we do face the reality of aging, it is with an anxiety so ferocious we sometimes don't want to discuss it or think about it. We equate growing old with losing things we value. In our twenties we start fretting about losing our youthful, smooth skin. In our thirties we must exercise continually, maniacally, to keep the firm body of our twenties. In our forties we think our eyes are going, our hair, our teeth, our sexual desire. We say things to our children such as, "I pray to God the time won't come when you have to put me in a home." Growing old fills us with dread once we convince ourselves that we've seen the best of our youth. And retirement means to far too many people a termination, a stopping, the end of the road. Even people who are fortunate enough to continue working into their seventies become frustrated, saying, "I can't do what I used to do." Retirement, we have sadly come to believe, is a limitation, a forced leap from the comfortable and familiar into a joyless nothingness.

Why have we departed so far from the Oriental reverence for the elderly? Why are the older members of our society not sought out and valued for their wisdom and their experience? Why is it that we let the vast experience of our elders go to waste in rocking chairs? Why do we view retirement as an end, a termination, leaving everything behind but not heading toward something? Why is the idea of growing old so dreaded? Why do we see aging as hopeless and negative?

Aging is a fact of life, neither intrinsically detrimental nor a negative stage of our development. Just as the sun comes up in the East each day, just as we must have food and drink, just as we need sleep, just as we find loving relationships and have children, so we all grow old. And we grow old with the idea that growing old is bad. Why is this? The sun's rising is good, indisputably. Certainly, having children is good, sleeping is good, and eating is good (up to a point). We have trouble, though, thinking in a positive way about aging. But aging is not bad in itself; aging is a series of physical and emotional changes taking place in our bodies and in our attitudes. Aging is another part of our development, a continuation of the changes that occur when we grow from babies into children, from children to teenagers, and from teenagers to adults. At these times of development, these transition periods, we change position. The teenager's position changes immensely from the earlier years of childhood, a time of relative stasis, of security. Teenagers' bodies and social lives change in dramatic upheavals, bringing fear and insecurity to many of them. From teen to adult, one's position changes again, rather dramatically, the world of responsibility closing in on the teen years they begin to say were carefree, all the problems of hormonal changes suddenly forgotten. At this point in our development, the reaching of "maturity," we choose to claim that we've lost our youth. Apparently, many of us feel that young is synonymous with carefree, or worse, irresponsible.

Aging brings new changes of position—physically, socially, financially, mentally. There are compensations for many of our aging changes—eyeglasses, hearing aids, pacemakers, pensions, age-segregated communities—but there are no compensations for the negative attitudes toward aging. Such negative attitudes are self-defeating. They are self-defeating because by accepting them we come to believe that old age is a feeble state. We hear of an old man who, because of disease, is too weak to get around much of his time, and we believe that the rocking chair is inevitable for everyone. We thus apply his situation anecdotally to the aging process and we fear for our future. When we accept such attitudes we tend, then, to let ourselves go. We don't take care of ourselves. We lose our health, we fall prey to disease, and we blame inevitability.

Scientific research today is disproving our historical, mythical view of old age. Being old is not synonymous with feebleness of body and mind.

Equating old with feeble is an outdated attitude begging for modernization in our day of new directions in healthy aging. Just as Oriental cultures convey value and self-worth to the elderly individual, so do their complex philosophical and meditative schools of thought provide surprisingly simple exercises in attitude-changing. Here's an example: From the sentence, Old people have no value to society, remove the tiny, two-letter word, no. Think about it. Such an easy exercise, yet when that small but immensely negative word is deleted, we may ponder an exciting future for ourselves: Old people have value to society. In fact, this moves beyond a word-play exercise when we reflect a moment to make a mental list of all those people in their seventies and eighties who play large roles in government, business, and entertainment. There are many young people who have no apparent value to society just as there are many old people too sick to continue as active participants. But a blanket declaration about all old people just won't do.

How about putting the exercise to this sentence: Retirement is the end of the road, the termination of a career. It's a common thought, yet more and more people are finding it easy to change that attitude so that today an entirely new prospect beckons them: Retirement is a different highway to travel, a new direction to follow, a beginning rather than an end.

Now for a big one: Older is not better. The transformation, Older is better, yields an idea certainly to be hoped, but is our little exercise superficial? Is it glib to say that growing older can be growing better? Research reported in these chapters, including scientific studies of nutrition, exercise, genetics, physiology, and mental health, show that we may realistically look forward to aging in good health. Changing our attitudes toward aging is an important, not a glib, part of the process. Making the effort to maintain our health is another.

Many, perhaps most, of the problems we have as we grow older develop because we do not pay attention to the basics of good health. We have been very careless about our health in Western society until the last couple of decades. We foolishly equated an unending supply of protein-rich red meat, luxurious automobiles to carry us to the corner grocery, and, yes, the cigarette, with prosperity and long life. Why, to be seen jogging or walking in the Fifties was to be thought to be poor, or, in some places, weird. Even now, after a barrage of fitness programs from books and videos, too many of us still become overweight or sedentary although common sense and science showed long ago that too much weight and too little activity are detrimental to good health. Many cases of diabetes, heart disease, and cancer could be prevented if we ate less, didn't smoke and got more exercise. By routinely working at staying healthy, trying to stay lean and active, and by practicing a positive, hopeful attitude, we can prevent most of the aches and pains of getting old. They are mostly anecdotal, anyway.

The Prejudice of Ageism

How do we define old age? Trying to get a consensus on the specific number of years denoting youth, middle age, and old age always proves interesting. "Young" doesn't present too much of a problem. People usually can agree it's from birth to 30 (well, some say 25) or 35, although these days some may want to stretch it to 40. Does youth end at 25 or at 40? That's a long spread of fifteen years . . . remember how much we change during our first fifteen years of life?

Well, then, how about middle age? Does it start at 40? Does it start at 25? Are we middleaged at 30? Are we middleaged at 50? 60? Many 60-year olds hardly think of themselves as old. Let's try old age. When does middle age become old age? 65? That's the official first year of old age as defined in the nineteen-thirties during the Depression years. But later, in the Seventies, age 62 replaced 65 for at least some Federal entitlement programs. Now there are moves to change to 66 or 67.

At age 67, some people plunge into crowded marinas for their windsurfing lessons. Some retire to nursing homes. At 70 some people lace up their new jogging shoes and run ten miles a day. Others at 40 collapse on their sofas, if not their rocking chairs, in front of the TV. But 40 is middle aged, no?

The effects of age vary from person to person. That point is easy to agree on, yet the sad fact remains that most of us commit "ageism," a term coined by gerontologist Robert Butler when he was director of the National Institute on Aging. We are all guilty of ageism when we assume that a person with gray hair has limited capabilities. We make assumptions about what he should or shouldn't do. The most obvious examples of ageism appear in advertising which perpetuates aging as a scourge, a curse that we can defeat not so much by using as by buying a plethora of creams and lotions and pills. Commercials appeal to our fears about aging: "Your eyes are the first place to betray your age. Let Clarins, France's premier skin care authority, come to the rescue." The rescue! We need the French to *save* us from the ravages of aging. "Does his hair give your age away?" is an especially clever one for it gives women the opportunity to blame their husbands for the passing of years. The Eighties have brought a somewhat more enlightened picture to us, such as an image of a gray-haired, round-bellied executive who gives his younger tennis partner a once-over on the court while his wife contentedly confides to the camera, "I'm so proud of him. He's not old at all." What she is really saying is "I want him to be young." She's so afraid of growing old that she's near hysterics. A recent ad for a skin cream reveals hysterical fear euphemistically transformed into a summons to battle when it says, "I don't intend to grow old gracefully . . . I intend to fight it every inch of the way."

Examples of ageism and myth appear daily in newspapers and magazines. The police "bust" of a poker parlor in Southern California provided readers of the Los Angeles Times a good laugh a year or two ago. The reporter carefully explained that the organizer of the illegal game was an elderly woman. She could not go immediately to the police station, she informed the arresting officers, because she needed first to go to the bathroom. Cute story. If the reporter wished to tickle his readers he might have stopped at that point. But he added a phrase after saying she needed to go to the bathroom: ". . . as old ladies are prone to do."

Let's assume he enjoyed his joke, but if he had taken the trouble of doing a minimal amount of research, he'd have found no biological evidence that shows old ladies are more apt to need the bathroom than 20-year olds of either sex, when busted by the police. The reporter was just another victim of anecdote, not to mention journalistic sloppiness.

In the height of the oil crisis, a newspaper story described a march by members of the Gray Panthers organization who were protesting high gasoline prices. The author implied that all old people have canes, hearing aids and Dr. Scholl comfort shoes along with them on their marches. Even worse, he wrote, "It was remarkable that some members of the crowd were able to complete the six and one-half block march, for it was obvious that their feet were killing them."

It is one thing for myth and anecdotal belief to provide, however mistakenly, a good laugh in a news story; when age prejudice is responsible for making health care decisions, elderly people are cruelly, if not primitively, treated at the hands of medical practitioners. Take the situation of a 65-year old woman whose gums are badly infected with periodontal disease. For whatever reasons—poverty, ignorance, a life of poor dental care—her teeth are on the verge of coming out of their sockets. Her dentist weighs his choices: total, expensive mouth rehabilitation or a clackety set of dentures. Money plays a big part in his decision. He's had his eye on a spiffy catamaran for this summer's toy. The woman can't afford the costly gum reconstruction and buying dentures will even be a hardship for her, he knows, but she can manage monthly payments for a couple of years. Getting his payment will prove easier with the dentures and, hell, she's an old lady who probably won't live much longer. Why go through all that mouth rehab?

The dentist has committed ageism. He has based his decision on the lady's age. He should have based it on the state of her periodontal disease and on whether rehabilitation of her gums appeared feasible, just as he would have done had his patient been 35 years old. Decisions about medical treatment must consider the age of a person, but they must consider far more than age. A 65-year old lady might live another thirty years and thirty years with one's own teeth are better than thirty years with dentures. Anyone with dentures will agree. Many of the pleasures of eating are sacrificed with the wearing of dentures.

Ageism and financial restraint have been responsible, in the last twenty years, for the institutionalization of many old people who may have fared better outside of nursing homes. Many young and middleaged people assume their old parents need to be taken care of and the old parents begin to think the same way. In the last twenty years, family responsibility for aging parents gave way to social responsibility, otherwise known as "government" or Medicare. There have been all too many sad stories about people pushed into nursing homes simply because government funds will pay for nursing home care or at least a good part of it. If the same people choose to stay in their own homes, they wouldn't be able to afford the medical care they need. This state of things has changed somewhat since 1980. We the people, so the story comes down from Washington, mandated a decline in government's social role. Sociologists and gerontologists are busy proclaiming the new era for family responsibility. It's nothing new. What was new in history, beginning only in the 1930s, was government responsibility. For five thousand years prior to that, families took care of their own. It just may be that the short-lived era of social responsibility will now decline and that family responsibility is the answer for many problems of our sick elderly people but the abrupt change in government's role, since 1980, has deprived many thousands of people of all ages of medical care.

Science Dispels Aging Myths

The fact is, we are just now emerging from the dark ages with respect to our knowledge of aging. Gerontology is a new science. It is just in our century that people have begun to live long enough to be considered elderly, or that sufficient numbers of elderly people have warranted a serious research effort. Before the twentieth century, family responsibility may have been the way for the support of old people but families simply did not have to care for their parents for very long. At the beginning of the nineteenth century life expectancy in the United States was 35 years. At the beginning of the twentieth century it had risen to 47. By the 1980s it had stretched to 74. Another myth of our day, similar to our society's belief that at age 65 we should sit in a rocking chair, is that elderly people, grandparents and great-grandparents used to be a very common element in family life. But aging researchers are now telling us that only in the twentieth century has it been likely for grandparents and grandchildren to get to know each other. In the past not many people survived to be grandparents for many years. If you were among the fifty percent who lived past age 35, your chances of seeing 45 or 50 decreased proportionately.

Our century has witnessed a booming acceleration of change—changes in education so that it became widespread, changes in production so that we are nonchalant about technological "miracles," changes in medicine such as the defeat of most infectious diseases, and a dramatic change in the numbers of elderly people. In 1900 only about four percent of the United States population was older than 65; now eleven or twelve percent are older than that. In forty or fifty years, it is expected, one in six Americans will be over 65. In actual numbers of people that is a jump, a leapfrog, from three million people in 1900 to fifty-five million in the year 2050. This acceleration in the numbers of the elderly coupled to the now aging post-World War II baby boom takes responsibility for the serious beginnings of aging research, for aging is now an economic question. Demographers seem to enjoy frightening the wits out of us with statistics showing that each of us will have to pay, in the year 2020, one-third of the nursing care costs of an old person. There being fifty-five million people over 65, they say, will mean allocations of our health care finances on a massive scale. Old people, through Social Security and Medicare, already receive twenty-seven percent of the national annual budget. Isn't it alarming, the Census Bureau writers ask, that more and more of the budget will go to caring for our elderly? But aren't we committing ageism when we assume that all those old people will require health care? Won't there be a continuation of changes in medical care, in personal health habits, and in new miracles brought by genetic technology?

New studies and research efforts are dispelling many unscientific, historically common notions about the elderly. Probably the most basic truth that gerontologists have learned in the last twenty years is that aging and disease are not the same. Aging is not a disease; it cannot be "cured." Of course, this is not to say that the elderly are free from disease. That is sadly not the case . . . yet. Old age is a time of increased susceptibility to disease and the demographic changes in our aging society are causing profound repercussions in the health care delivery systems of the developed world. This is true not only because of the greater numbers of people who need care, but also because the health care requirements of elderly people and their responses to treatment are slightly, sometimes greatly, different from younger people's. Defining these requirements and responses presents problems in health care simply because in many cases the data has not been gathered. Physicians are not always attuned to the differences between their young and old patients.

The good news, science is telling us, is that old age is not necessarily filled with disease. Old age can be a time of good health. This is what scientists have been learning and what is pointing our direction now: Aging cannot be stopped but it can be a time of good health. We are discovering ways to make old age less susceptible to the ravages of disease. There is no fountain of youth but there is a fountain of health and finding it is quite within our power. Science, by disproving anecdotal belief, is allowing us to overcome our fear of aging. It is not an oversimplification to say that now we may age hopefully and healthfully.

Do people really live longer today than in earlier times? Yes and no. The terms "life expectancy" and "life span" have different meanings. Life expectancy today is somewhat higher than 73 for men and 78 for women. (Ardent political arguments notwithstanding, there is something biologically different in men and women—hormones, for one thing.) But what does life expectancy mean? Does it mean that since I am a man I can expect to live until 73 and suddenly go out like a light bulb? Does it mean that I as a woman, expecting to live until 78, will get five years over my husband? No. Life expectancy is really a statistic, used primarily by insurance companies and government agencies which deal in budgets for large groups of people. It means that half of all men are dead by the age of 73; half survive to exceed that age. And fifty percent of women live longer than 78; fifty percent die before.

Life expectancy, then, is important for judging the well-being of the whole society. As a planning tool, it is statistically necessary. As mere statistics though, life expectancy figures tell a person nothing about his individual aging prospects or his life span. It is life span, not life expectancy, which is important to an individual, his life span being the age at which he dies. If I die at age 50 my life span is fifty years. And I am a member of the unlucky half of the population that sets the life expectancy figures for everyone. I am among that fifty percent dead before age 73.

The potential life span of us human beings, *homo sapiens*, hasn't changed in fifty thousand years. Our species can individually live from 70 to 115, the oldest accurately recorded age. That range of years is our biological life span, our possible longevity if disease or accident leaves us untouched. Some insects live a day or two, most dogs live between ten and seventeen years, and some trees survive for centuries. As species go, we, with 70 to 115 years, are a rather long-lived one. And nowadays we can expect to live out our biological life span when just one hundred and eighty years ago the expectation was thirty-five years. What happened? Why are we able to grow old now? The members of our medical profession would have us believe our new longevity is all their doing. For due to the discovery and widespread use of antibiotics and immunizations, physicians bask in our esteemed gratitude. But the fact is, the physicians must share the credit with the garbagemen. A dramatic reason for our doubled life expectancy, aside from medical advancements, is vast improvements in sanitation and hygiene. Just imagine New York City in the middle of the nineteenth century when the horse and buggy provided the primary mode of transportation. There was pollution of a different order from our present chemical problems. The biological pollution was scattered on the streets. And it was a form of pollution that attracted flies—carriers of infectious diseases. And this was not all. To feed all those horses it was necessary to maintain huge storehouses of grain. Where there are stores of grain, there are rats. Rats carry flies. In such an environment cholera, dysentery, and plague spread easily.

But immunization against childhood diseases is also responsible for our long lives. Diphtheria was one of the biggest killers, taking many children, as well as entire families, in the early part of the twentieth century. Religious sanctions for having large families were always due, in large measure, to the fact that you needed reserves. That was a fact in our young country a hundred years ago and it is still a fact in many parts of the world.

Disturbing reports these last few years relate that many parents are not taking their children to receive vaccinations. Is it that people forget about diphtheria and polio because of the myth that these diseases are defeated? Or is it due to the high cost of vaccinations? The scientific fact is that no one can say with certainty that a particular virus is extinct simply because there have not been any cases of infection in fifteen or twenty years. The way to make sure is to immunize; epidemics could break out again. Government may be short-sighted, seeing the present need to be thrifty but not the future danger to public health, and a family may not be able to afford the high cost of a vaccination. One can only hope that such preventive health care will one day be everyone's birthright, as it is in some northern European countries, some of which have a higher standard of living than the budget-conscious U.S.A.

Such scientific research as the Baltimore Longitudinal Study of Aging, a major data collection endeavor by the National Institute on Aging, is truly consigning our ageistic negative image of elderly people to the dark ages. The Baltimore study is ambitiously following the lives of a thousand people whose ages range from 20 to 96. Among the well-documented, anecdote-shattering news: Sexual pleasure does not decrease in old age, indeed, it may become better. Women may find increased enjoyment in sexual activities as they age, and men seem, for the most part, to maintain the same level of sexual activity throughout their lives. Personalities rarely change drastically with age; a cranky old man typically was a cranky young man. And if our elderly people are depressed, the cause is not inevitably due to growing old. Unfortunately, depression is the greatest mental health problem old people face and it is caused by our social conditions and by drugs, not by aging changes of the central nervous system.

Aging and the Fountain of Health

Up to now, ageism and advertising have given aging an ugly face and a rather huge segment of our economy devotes itself to products and potions purporting to cure wrinkles, age spots, and gray hair. If we lost our fear of aging, taking a more enlightened and hopeful view, and if we stopped buying those products (most of them useless), our economy might take a nose dive of deficit-worsening proportions. True, our social deficit would improve. Changes are already underway in mass marketing and in advertising reflecting the shifting of our median age. The baby boom of the late Forties and the Fifties mass-produced a generation glorified by advertising. Now, it appears, as the baby boom youngsters turn into a middleaged boom and then into a geriatric swell, the marketing of products will continue to be directed toward them. Already, advertising includes older models, and the median age in the United States is over 30. It is predicted that by the year 2020 there will be as many people over age 37 as under 37.

One suspects hopefully that physical characteristics of older people—wrinkles and gray hair—will become desirable as society's median age increases. One is also hopeful that age itself will gain the respect it deserves. Neither is possible without the good health of elderly people. Staying healthy is the way to look good, too, and a myth many of us still believe is that old people should not exercise. We've been conditioned to believe that once you're old, you can't or shouldn't exert yourself physically. It is certainly true that a person at age 50 should not attempt to run ten miles early one Saturday morning if he hasn't jogged in twenty years, but then the same precaution applies to a 25-year old who's out of shape, doesn't it? Gerontologists are learning that old people gain strength from physical exercise in much the same way that young people do, again, disproving anecdotal ageism. Old people, like young people, can improve their health by regular exercise, although middleaged and older people don't show health improvement as rapidly as young people who take up exercise, because the body's metabolism (its functioning in general) has slowed down a little in middle and old age. The slowdown in metabolism is also the reason why many people gain a "middleaged spread." As we age we're not burning up as much food as when we're young. We don't need as much and we should cut down on the amount of food we eat as we age.

More and more magazines these days display "health awareness" themes with articles about the benefits of exercise and proper nutrition. These articles are directed to people over the age of 30 and this is a healthful trend—readers presumably are learning how to stay healthy. Too often, though, these publications include sensational ads and articles which prey on people's fears and perpetuate the negativism of ageism. Such ads promise the fountain of youth in capsules sent through the mail and paid for by credit cards. This is profiteering from ageism and it is a contemporary form of the hucksterism practiced on our frontier in the nineteenth century. In those days, tipsy salesmen hawked bottles of curative elixirs; now they sell superoxide dismutase (SOD). "Take SOD three times a day," say the ads, "and be youthful again." One company even claims that SOD *stops* the aging process.

Well, SOD is, in fact, a wonderful chemical. It is an enzyme made right in our own bodies. It protects the membranes of our cells from molecular troublemakers like superoxide. But eating SOD itself won't give us more of this beneficial enzyme. When we take nutrients, food of any kind, our digestive systems break them down into their basic components, amino acids, that we can use. A lump of SOD taken orally doesn't remain SOD; in digestion we break it up into forms no longer resembling SOD. And those forms don't help us produce SOD more than anything else we eat. To say that a capsule of SOD will make us youthful is like saying we'll grow a watermelon by eating watermelon seeds. Beware of those who would sell the fountain of youth. It's not for sale.

Chapter 2

The Fundamental
Molecule of Life

We human beings and all other life on earth are the physical results of microscopic bits of nucleic acid and chemical reactions. The nucleic acid, which contains all the information for our physical development, is in the primary cell—the egg and sperm. We are just like a seed at that stage and, like plants, we need food, air, and water. DNA, a microscopic bit of nucleic acid, safely locked up and guarded in the innermost structure of a cell (the nucleus) passes our inheritance to us from our parents. It contains our genes, dictating our potential structure, strengths, and weaknesses. The interaction of this inheritance with the environment we are born into directs our development, our growth, and then, our aging.

Understanding most of today's research about aging requires some general knowledge of DNA—what it is, how it works, and, sometimes, how it fails to work. Contemporary theories of aging, the subject of the next chapter, become clearer when approached with some rudiments of genetics. We believe that the best introduction to such an understanding of DNA, genetics, and the broader field of molecular biology is a description of our world's newest industry—biotechnology.

We are living and aging in a particularly important time for scientific research—molecular biology is yielding up its mysterious secrets to scientists and from the biotechnology which results, there is a strong possibility that we may age with more hope and with better health than past generations. Science has discovered the physical basis of inheritance in the gene, the mechanism which determines the characteristics of all living things. Genetics, the branch of molecular biology which studies inheritance, provides previously undreamed of possibilities for retarding the degenerative effects of old age. An example: One of the latest marvels is the manufacture of tissue plasminogen activator (TPA), a protein occurring naturally in our bodies which dissolves blood clots. Clots can form in the bloodstream when circulation is impeded and they can block blood flow to the heart muscles which not only causes heart attacks but also adds to their severity. In seconds, an injection of TPA can clear the blocked blood vessel, providing not only survival but also a greater chance that serious heart damage will not result.

The most important thing about TPA is the speed with which it works. For several years, a drug called streptokinase has been used for dissolving clots in coronary heart disease, but its administration (by catheter through an artery in the groin) means that its effects are realized in minutes. Heart attack damage occurs rapidly, though, and minutes are not good enough. TPA works in seconds and recombinant DNA research made it a reality.

There is no question that the blueprints within our cells will unfold a future full of marvels for mankind. But perhaps it is better to say that one is hopeful such marvels will be realized. Molecular biology comes with controversy, opening the doors to the possibility of changing life as we know it, as well as improving it. Beyond the doors, in the unknown corridors, there are unanswered questions not only for science and medicine, but also for religion and ethics.

The description of deoxyribonucleic acid (DNA) by James Watson and Francis Crick in 1952 was one of those milestones in the history of discovery—as dazzling for our time as Galileo's vision of the solar system was for his. DNA is the fundamental molecule of life. Molecular biology is the branch of biology explaining life at the most elementary level—the joining of molecules to form living organisms such as bacteria and people. Genetics is a grandchild of Charles Darwin, for it illustrates the mechanics of evolution. Watson and Crick won the immediate praise and esteem of humanity, unlike Darwin, whose work was and continues to be a center of controversy. Perhaps it can be said that the notoriety of his theories of evolution and natural selection opened the way for the ready acceptance of the mechanics of the genes. At any rate, DNA is the essence of natural selection and of the evolution of life. Through inheritance, DNA determines what our genes will be, just as it determines the genes of our livestock and the genes of our agricultural produce. Inheritance of "good genes" or "bad genes" is responsible for adaptation and change in species. In a basic way, genes are central to the success or failure of any living thing.

Genetics and the (Near) Future

Molecular biology and genetics are really still in their infancy. At this stage, scientists are just observing; they are describing molecular details, but they don't yet know how all the details work. What they know is enough that we may glimpse a different world. Molecular biology has the potential power to give us all the energy we need to make our world comfortable. It promises abundance in agriculture so that, for the first time in history, enough food can be produced to go round. It promises ways to clean our air, land, and water. It promises the demise of birth defects, the delay of age-onset diseases, and the prolonging of the good health that we associate with youth.

Scientists and oil companies are exploring the realms of biology for ways to replace the earth's finite supply of fossil fuels—our oil and gas. Plants convert the energy from sunlight into chemical energy by photosynthesis which manufactures sugar. Plants also convert energy into gases. One of these gases is oxygen which, of course, is responsible for the creation of animals and man. Biology holds the key to our mimicking plants; scientists can learn the secrets of photosynthesis and put them to work making our energy. Perhaps soon we can install a small box of photosynthesizing battery cells on our roofs, capturing our sun's energy to run our homes and saying adieu to the problems of fossil fuels. We've already started doing this, but we're using a primitive cumbersome apparatus called a solar panel.

Another possibility is the growing of fuel in agricultural fields, "biomass" technology. Already, such plants as the rubber tree and its family are promising abundant oil. We can learn genetically to improve the output of oil from such plants, multiplying their individual oil-producing capacities, and what's more, we can genetically adapt them to grow almost anywhere on earth. It is not far fetched to imagine putting vast areas of the earth—far north or far south, or arid lands, now unproductive—to use as farmland for plants genetically developed just for such areas.

Genetics can provide us with the ways to multiply our food supply. Man has been manipulating animal and plant species for thousands of years, breeding through hybridization those specimens which yield the most and the best food. We have developed many species of plants and animals because of their useful qualities, thus replacing natural selection with artificial or human selection. We select and breed cows which give the most milk and we select chickens which lay the most eggs. Now it is possible to create wholly new species, say, beef cattle which need a fraction of the feed now necessary to bring a bull to market. It is now possible to create a species of corn which not only yields many times the ears of a typical corn stalk today, but by mixing its genes with bacteria that make fertilizer, we can eliminate the high cost of fertilizer.

Attempts to genetically engineer plants and micro-organisms have raised concerns about potential dangers to the environment and to the public health. Lawsuits have been filed and experimentation has, in some cases, been halted. The concern is due to the fact that in the past, the introduction of new agricultural practices proved hazardous—the use of the insecticide DDT, for example. But the expected economic and environmental benefits from biotechnology are tremendous. By splicing certain genes with resistance to insects into food plants it will be possible to increase the world's food supply and the great hope is that such improved plant stock will then mean less use of toxic pesticides and fungicides. It is these chemicals which have constituted the real danger from agribusiness, and genetic manipulation may make them obsolete.

Of course, concern is raised too, that genetically engineered plants may prove toxic themselves. But hybridization of plants has been practiced for centuries and, once in a while, poisonous plants have indeed resulted. Up to now, however, hybrid techniques have been rather willy-nilly, usually with little or no knowledge of the possibility of danger. With genetics, the hybridization no longer must be random; specific objectives may be pursued by specific molecular materials.

Bacteria have always played a large role in life on earth. They help us and they hinder us; they bring us disease, but life without them is not possible. Their potential role is expanding through the technology learned from molecular biology. Man is now creating bacteria to "eat" oil spills. Only a step further are bacteria which will remove pollutants from the air or even from our factories, the root of the problem, so that there is no harmful discharge into the air or into our rivers. Imagine benign bacteria genetically developed to cannibalize the cavity producing bacteria in our mouths. And then imagine the same talented creatures snacking on sugar and plaque, keeping our teeth clean for us like snails in a fish bowl—keeping our gums free from disease. Imagine a band of bacteria in our stomachs, not only aiding our digestion, as they always have, but producing vitamins for us—perhaps much or all of our vitamin needs. Of course, we would have to eat something to nourish the bacteria, say, paper or wood. Bacteria may consume our wastes and garbage for us in the future, making sludge and landfills memories of our barbaric past. They may dig our mines, ending the dangers for human miners of cave-ins and gas leaks.

These days, scientific journals report weekly the developments in biotechnology—bacteria which can make medicines, insecticides, chemical livestock feed, you name it. Bacteria are making human insulin for us now, in much the same way they have supplied us with cheese throughout history. We can create the bacteria we need—genetics gives us the tools.

Another way that genetics will help us age in better health is through prenatal diagnosis of disease or susceptibility to disease, already in use for several years in such procedures as amniocentesis (analyzing an unborn child's genes from a drop of fetal fluid) and chorionic biopsy. One of the first diseases to be diagnosed in this way was sickle cell anemia, recognizable because of the knowledge that a DNA cleavage enzyme, MST II, cuts out a single fragment from a strand of genes when the blood cell condition is present. Thalassemia, a blood cell disease found often in the Mediterranean area of the world, has been reduced because of molecular prenatal diagnosis. Other procedures, too, the use of synthetic oligonucleotides and various genetic markers, are valuable in confirming genetic defects in fetuses when family history indicates such a probability.

But controversial questions ensue: Will diagnostic results be used by insurance companies and employers to discriminate against hapless possessors of defective genes?

Monoclonal antibodies—used for diagnostic purposes, experimental treatments for cancer, and in vaccines—were developed by immunologists Cesar Milstein and Georges

Kohler in 1974 when they combined a blood cell with a cancerous cell. What they invented was a cell with the ability to produce a defense against cancer and with the ability to divide indefinitely, an improvement over the immune capability of human cells. Advances like these have made experiments possible for correcting genetic defects such as treatment for adenosine deaminase deficiency, the disease of the so called "bubble children," and for patients with Lesch-Nyhan syndrome. These developments are also controversial, raising ethical questions: Are scientists trying to play God (or Mother Nature) by changing human chemistry in their repair or replacement of defective genes? The debate has been joined by Congress, whose Office of Technology Assessment in 1985 distinguished between gene therapy affecting somatic cells or affecting germ cells. Correcting defects in somatic cells is one thing, according to Congress's report, and differs hardly at all from traditional medical procedure since genetic change is confined to the patient at hand. Changing genes in germ cells, however, represents a brand new step in medicine since it is the germ cells which carry inheritance to our offspring. Germ cell therapy affects not only the patient at hand but also all the future generations of his family. Congress held off on sanctioning germ cell gene therapy, citing a lack of public ethical acceptance.

Genetics will change medical care fundamentally. Although we cannot do away with disease altogether, it is becoming more and more likely that we will learn to buttress our own disease-fighting force, the immune system. Thus, cancer might go the way of polio and we just might cure the common cold at long last—or never get one at all. By strengthening our immune system, by genetically protecting ourselves from age-onset problems like diabetes and cardiovascular disease, we will leap again in life expectancy. It is possible to consider living out a life span of 115 years. And assuming we make the most of our knowledge of biology, we can be hopeful of living out our life span in good health.

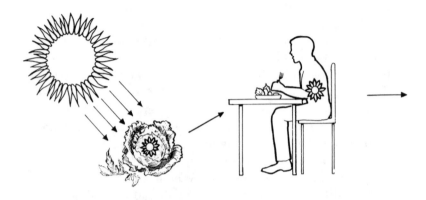

Figure 1   Solar-powered human cells: Plants collect energy from the sun, providing carbohydrate in our diet. This nutrient is broken down into molecules of glucose which react with oxygen . . .

The Energy of Living and Aging

We live and age because of chemical energy. Atoms react with each other biochemically not only to form structures (such as a leaf or a baby), but also to make energy flow so that growth and change can occur. For our world and everything in it, energy begins in the sun and flows through the chemistry of life on earth. Just as oxygen reacts with gasoline to make a flame, oxygen reacts with sugar inside our cells to provide energy to make us live. The sugar (carbohydrate) comes to us by way of green plants whose leaves collect the energy from the sun and convert it to foodstuffs which we then gather and eat. Inside our cells we have little power plants of oxidation, the mitochondria, which efficiently convert molecules of glucose (containing energy from the sun which we have digested) into yet another form of chemical energy that we can use. The final product of the mitochondria is a molecule

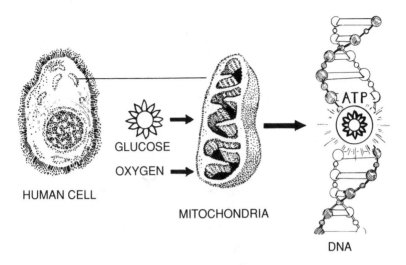

GLUCOSE

OXYGEN

HUMAN CELL

MITOCHONDRIA

ATP

DNA

. . . inside the cells' power plants, the mitochondria, to form ATP, a molecule of highly concentrated energy used to spark DNA and other chemical reactions of the body.

called adenosine triphosphate (ATP) and it supplies energy for most of the chemical reactions in the body.

It is this energy, sent by the sun and stored for us in plants so that we can convert it for our needs, which sparks our admirable molecules of DNA to unravel hereditary information into instructions for structural growth. In the manner of a twisted, doubled telephone cord that is pulled straight, DNA serves as a medium for the communication of vital information—sex, build, early (or late) baldness, eye color, degree of hirsuteness, disease susceptibilities. Each cell in the human body contains DNA and all our genes arrayed on forty-six chromosomes. Periodically, enzymes cleave or unzip the double helix of DNA so that replication is possible. And so, when the cells divide, DNA is in each nucleus. Its message, the instructional blueprint for the construction and the maintenance of the body, leaves the cell nucleus by transcribing itself onto the more expendable ribonucleic acid (RNA) which exits the nucleus. DNA is far too valuable to leave the security of the nucleus of the cell; somewhat like a queen bee, it stays in place where the body's workers come to receive their orders.

Recombinant DNA technology really is quite simple in theory, but in practice it is painstakingly precise. Insulin is now more widely available to people who need it because science discovered how to instruct rapidly reproducing bacteria (the now famous *Escherichia coli*) to produce it. By splicing a sequence of DNA that codes for insulin into the bacteria's genes, the mutated bacteria unwittingly churn out the hormone in any quantity desired.

A Digression on Proteins, Amino Acids, and the Genetic Code

RNA transcribes the hereditary information in the gene which translates into instructions for the construction of proteins. Then the proteins create us and all our bodily functions— including our ability to reproduce and pass our DNA on to our children. Actually, DNA is made of four "nucleotide bases," adenosine (from ATP), thymidine, guanine, and cytosine; to form DNA, they pair by electrical attraction just like magnets and metal. Adenosine always pairs with thymidine; guanine pairs with cytosine. When a geneticist reads a strand of DNA with three bases as "AGA," the sequence of opposite bases on the paired strand is "TCT." It is the individual arrangements of these pairings that make us physically different from other human beings. Our DNA is our individually coded sequence, and no one else has an exact copy of it . . . unless we have an identical twin. Sequences of the pairings, hundreds of them at a stretch, have become known as genes.

Sometimes, disease susceptibility results from "point mutations" in the sequence of base pairs—a fact that provides us an opportunity to forestall or prevent disease, now that the

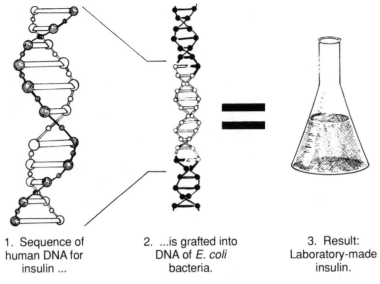

1. Sequence of
human DNA for
insulin ...

2. ...is grafted into
DNA of *E. coli*
bacteria.

3. Result:
Laboratory-made
insulin.

Figure 2   Recombinant DNA: Technology puts bacteria to
work for us. Certain bacteria which rapidly reproduce, such
as *Escherichia coli*, can actually manufacture large quantities
of insulin when the DNA-coded insulin blueprint is spliced
into their genes.

*complex workings of genetics is being decoded. For example,
many people with emphysema have a deficiency of a particular
protein whose function it is to protect the lungs from environmental damage. The protein deficiency is due to a difference of
one base in these people's genes—a point mutation. By extrac-
ting and analyzing the sequential strand from the chromosome
of a person, and by finding the defective gene, a geneticist can
predict emphysema for that person who, armed with the knowledge, is advised to take preventive measures such as not
smoking, or moving to a relatively unpolluted part of the
world. Soon, no doubt, a genetic laboratory somewhere will
synthesize the actual protein, and manufacture it (as they have
done with insulin) so that it can be given as a drug.*

*It is thought that a cell probably has about one hundred
thousand genes, the functions of most of them still unknown.*

Around one thousand have been identified, but the process, called "gene mapping," is accelerating. We have learned that it's not only little girls who are made of sugar and spice and everything nice: DNA and RNA are partly sugar and partly phosphate and there are at least three forms of RNA. "Messenger" RNA is the one which has copied DNA for the structure of a protein and feeds the information into the cellular factories called ribosomes. "Ribosomal" RNA puts all the chemicals in place for a reaction to occur and then it assembles finished products, proteins, from bits of amino acid. "Transfer" RNA picks up these bits of amino acids throughout the cell and delivers them to the ribosomes. Every three nucleotide bases along a row of RNA make the code for one amino acid; this is what is called the genetic code. Just as DNA is a row of nucleotides, a protein is a row of amino acids linked together like a chain. The row of amino acids is a replica of the row of nucleotide bases but it has a different chemical form. Technically, only a relatively small portion of DNA is used for specifying the amino acid sequence and the function of only small stretches of sequences is known. Sequences containing code are known as exons, and non-coding intervening sequences are known as introns. In passing information to RNA, only DNA's exons are transcribed.

And why is the chemical form of amino acids important? There are twenty-two of them and they are the products of the food that we have digested, although some are also made by our cells. The genetic code in messenger RNA assembles proteins by putting together these chains of amino acids. The particular combinations of the acids along the chain for making particular proteins are the information in the genetic code.

Some sensational magazine articles try to convince people to buy and eat nucleic acids, just as they try to sell SOD. The articles say that eating nucleic acids will boost one's levels of RNA or DNA, keep the body working in tip-top shape, retard aging, and so forth, and typically, the articles are followed by ads showing how and where to purchase them. Don't believe such nonsense; any nutrient a person swallows will be broken *down by digestive enzymes and then reformed to make chains of nucleotides and amino acids. Eating RNA will not cause more RNA. Nucleic acid is a very personal thing.*

Molecular Medicine

How do genetic mutations happen? Molecules, life's building blocks, form when complementary atoms join. A molecule of water (H_2O) contains two hydrogen atoms and one oxygen atom. When scientists talk of "free radicals" they are speaking of stray atoms which have not found complementary atoms and so have not become part of a molecule. In the course of its helter-skelter travels, a stray atom can bump into the DNA molecule and cause an accident, a mutation, or error which changes the sequence of the code. Harmful agents like nicotine, ultraviolet radiation and nitrites likewise cause mutations in our DNA. One aging theory, in fact, says that the reason we grow old is the accumulation of such mistakes over a lifetime. Other free radicals can tear holes in the cell membranes, effectively destroying cells since the contents then spill out. The praises that one hears of Vitamin C are justified; much scientific evidence seems to show that Vitamin C assists in destroying free radicals before they harm the cells.

Scientists are on the verge of genetic discoveries which will enable physicians to alter their thrust from treatment of symptoms to actual prevention of disease, for they will possess the tools to fight disease on a molecular level. One already hears these days of "turning on" specific genes which can "turn off" specific diseases. Many scientists are looking for ways to turn off oncogenes which are precursors of cancer—mutations thought to be caused by radiation, chemicals, viruses, and other DNA-altering agents.

Viruses plague mankind and animals as virulent pathogens, bringing us illnesses ranging from the flu, to brain disorders such as encephalitis, to immune deficiencies such as AIDS. Today, many scientists believe viruses are also the initiators of many cancers. Genetics, through the new recombinant DNA technology, holds the hope for our finally taking the upper hand over viruses. A virus harms us by commandeering our own DNA and replicating itself with our molecular machinery. When it sneaks past our initial defenses of mucus (sneezing or coughing), the wavy, hairlike cilia on the cell's membranes, and the attacks by the white blood cells, it chews a hole through a cell wall and makes its way through the interior cytoplasm to the nucleus. Entering, the virus substitutes its DNA for ours and we thus produce new viruses at such a rate that the cell bursts, spilling out self-manufactured pathogens which take over other cells, repeating the process until we're acutely ill, with millions of viruses to be reckoned with.

Many viruses give us a protracted battle while others elude the immune system's defense altogether, quietly nourishing themselves at our expense for many years, becoming harmful, seemingly at their own pleasure. Many age-onset degenerative illnesses besides cancer (including coronary heart disease, organic brain syndrome, arthritis, diabetes, ulcers, and emphysema) may very well have viral origins. Up to now, drugs and vaccines have been of little help, but genetically-engineered vaccines are rapidly being produced with the knowledge of the workings of DNA. Genetics opens the possibility of retarding aging by giving us ways to produce defense against these diseases of old age. Laboratories around the world are competing, as a matter of fact, to create synthetic antigens that resemble the receptors of pathogenic microorganisms which, when injected in the bloodstream, prepare the body's immune system to fight the real microorganism when it contacts it. Another possibility is to tinker molecularly with a pathogen, rewording its genetic code to remove its sting by causing a mutation that robs it of its virulence. Still another technique, well within science's capability now, is to artificially grow antibodies to a given virus

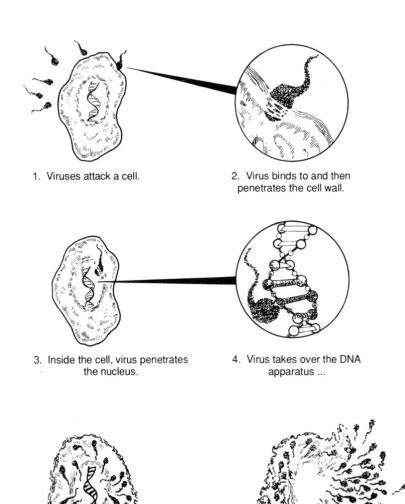

1. Viruses attack a cell.

2. Virus binds to and then penetrates the cell wall.

3. Inside the cell, virus penetrates the nucleus.

4. Virus takes over the DNA apparatus ...

5. ... and uses DNA for virus reproduction, usurping the cell's normal functions.

6. Virus-laden cell bursts and dies; new viruses rush to invade other cells and repeat the cycle.

Figure 3   How a virus commandeers a human cell.

and use them in a vaccine, allowing a headstart for immune defense.

Genetics for Profit?

Physicians nowadays have to be aware of a proliferation of drugs and diagnostic tools that may become available and then be obsolete before their use is widespread. CAT scan radiation photography, only recently the rage for spotting tumors, is already giving way to the new techniques of ultrasound and magnetic resonance imaging. Technology from genes and microchips are taught in medical schools now, but our future physicians are also learning that technology is a tool rather than a magic cure. There are other forces, to be sure, besides genetic manipulation.

It is hard to imagine gene mapping and recombinant DNA providing answers to why hopeful attitudes are often curative in the most puzzling illnesses. Physicians know that so called "terminal illnesses" are sometimes turned around more by a patient's emotional state than by any technological breakthrough. An individual's will to fight off a disease seems to somehow marshall the body's defenses in ways that technology can never equal. One can be hopeful indeed, about the future of medicine if physicians and patients maintain respect both for technology and for those mysteries of our own curative abilities.

Very questionable, however, is our historical penchant for putting our research money into projects promising financial profit rather than basic and applied knowledge. It has been pointed out in scientific journals that the best geneticists today have ties with industry. Big business lures scientists with greater rewards than we taxpayers are willing to offer them in our government research programs. What this means is that decisions for applying genetic discovery are more influenced by a corporate board than by society as a whole, and a corporate board's primary concern is distributing dividends to stockholders. Isn't this the wrong way to go about scientific and medical research? A technique may be found for preventing a birth defect only so long as the birth defect is prevalent enough to ensure wide sales of the technique and large profits. But what about the rare birth defect that strikes only a few babies? Will our system of financial incentives ignore those babies?

The future of genetics is too important to be decided solely by businessmen. Likewise, the decisions for using our genetic knowledge are too important to be left to our scientists. Our educational system must try to teach molecular biology so that an informed democratic society can make its own decisions for using its new knowledge. The future will see the unfolding of many more secrets: How does DNA discriminate among all the functions of the body? How does it instruct proteins to build the parts of the body? These are central questions in biology today. How do the cells differentiate and know their functions? How does an egg cell, joined by sperm, divide and keep dividing to create cells for building arms and legs, other cells to make a heart, a liver, breasts, a brain, hair, genitals, a tongue, a set of teeth, the skin, hormones, bones? Although no one knows the answer yet, it seems likely that the answer will soon be found and it will lead to the cure or prevention of our most dreaded diseases, for knowing the secret of cellular function will give us the key to correcting cellular malfunction such as cancer.

Other questions lie in the realm of the theories of aging. Is it errors in the synthesis of DNA that are responsible for aging? Is there a faulty, perhaps an innate, genetic mechanism leading to errors in the chromosomes which lead, in turn, to faulty protein construction, leading further to breakdowns in the body's metabolism? Are the errors caused by mutations from the daily assault from free radicals, a lifetime of wear and tear? Do the errors take place in DNA itself or do they occur in the process of transcription to RNA? Is there a genetic clock in the nucleus of each cell, ticking with regularity until we have developed and reproduced ourselves— serving evolution's objective and knowing then that it is time to wind down?

Chapter 3

Why Do We Age?

Ever since man became aware that he could ask questions about life—and more important, take actions to modify and improve his lot on earth—aging and death have been philosophical preoccupations. Why do we age? Does skin wrinkle and lose its elasticity because of chronic wear and tear on our bodies over the course of our lives? The ancient Greeks, knowledgeable about atoms and other particles, knew that human beings and all living things were prey to the elements of sun, rain, and wind which, over the course of many years, can destroy the integrity of physical matter. Certainly our own era in history testifies to environmental wear and tear. We are more acutely aware of the hazards in our environment than people of previous times because we have created asbestos, dioxin, ionizing radiation, and many other chemical pollutants which are dangerous not just to our skin, but also to all our cells—our entire molecular makeup. We are also aware that a lifetime of psychological stress bodes no less ill to our cardiovascular system than nicotine, caffeine, and a diet high in fats. Wear and tear affects the immune system also, chronic infection straining the body's defense and healing capacity, leaving it increasingly susceptible, as it ages, to more disease and injury.

Some people believe that a daily habit of sexual activity, a sort of wear and tear, shortens life, while others maintain that sex not only enriches life but prolongs it too. Alas, there's no scientific evidence for either viewpoint; the sexual theory of aging is more anecdotal than factual.

The wear and tear theory for the processes of aging, formally called the stochastic theory, cannot convincingly explain why one person reacts to environmental assault differently from another. Some cigarette smokers, of course, continue their pack a day habit well into their seventies or eighties. Some people recover from rheumatic heart disease and go on to participate in ten-mile jogging marathon competitions. Obviously, human beings come differently equipped to brave the elements of our world and so another theory, the genetic explanation of aging, allows for a built-in biological clock, specific not only for each species of living beings, but also for each member of the species. Adherents of the genetic theory say that each of us is programmed like a computer to perform certain functions, such as growing, reproducing, and dying. While we are performing these functions or living our lives, our biological clock ticks ineluctably toward a planned demise. DNA gives us genetic susceptibilities to certain ailments and diseases, so it is predestined that we will succumb to one of them. Every species of life on earth possesses its unique biological life span, human beings included. Our life span peaks at about 110 or 115 years, while many insects live only a day or two. Dogs live 10 to 18 years, while tortoises in the Galapagos Islands trudge over barren landscapes, eating and reproducing for 150 years or more. Giant trees in the California Sierra Mountains continue to grow and thrive for thousands of years. Why do some species of living things spend a short time on earth while others remain such a long time? Is there something in the genetic programs of the long-lived other species that we can somehow emulate in our own chromosomes?

A third major theory, the evolutionary theory of aging, envelops both the genetic and the environmental theories, arguing that both heredity and outside influences act in combination to ensure not only the propagation but also the improvement of each species. Individuals must age and die, according to this theory, so that the species may prosper.

But what is aging? It is not easy to pin down a definition

other than to list the obvious physical changes that occur to us as we grow old. Aging is not the same as disease. It can't be "cured." Some people age seemingly free from disease while others die from disease at a very young age. Many diseases accelerate the aging process and aging often leads to disease susceptibility. Everything and everyone ages and dies at rates according to inner constitution and outside hazards. A well built house of brick and mortar possesses more probability of surviving the onslaught of a hurricane than does a paperboard shack just as a healthy athlete who maintains physical training, keeps a regular schedule, and eats only the right amount of the right foods will probably resist a virus that causes havoc in a weaker person. But the brick and mortar home, if not renewed for, say, a hundred years, inevitably will suffer decay. Eventually, it may even fall under a strong storm. Our athlete's state of good health will one day fail him, too, leaving him open to viral infection.

Aging seems best defined as the body's gradual loss of function and organization. With the passage of time neither mortar nor collagen can maintain its original strength; both will give way to changes in structure. Since Albert Einstein's day, we have defined everything in our world as relative to something else; aging and time are no exceptions. Some people define aging as the specific slowdown in the body's cell division. Seen relative to an infant's development and growth, when cells divide like wildfire, this definition also is valid. In relation to the fact, however, that cells in different parts of the body slow their division at different rates and at different times, this definition of aging does not stand the test.

Can we say that our cells age? They usually divide to form "daughter" cells. Are these two completely new cells or are they really one "old" cell and one "young" cell? When we say that a giant redwood tree is over a thousand years old are we talking specifically about the dead part of the tree in the center of its trunk or are we talking about the new growth at the tip of its branches? Isn't the new growth only one year old? Aging is relative to time as we know and define time and to change as we know and define change. A bouncing ball does not bounce forever but only in relation to the material composing it and to the energy throwing it. Eventually, its material loses its elasticity—the ball wears out—and it won't bounce no matter how much energy propels it.

Ticking Away the Years

What really concerns us when we define aging, our own relativity to aging, are the changes that occur in us as we age and we can describe these changes: Our hair turns gray, it thins or maybe it falls out; our skin loses elasticity and it wrinkles; our muscles lose size and strength; our bones break more easily; our hearing levels change; we tire more quickly.

The genetic theory of aging holds that these changes are periodic occurrences in a life program charted in DNA's control center in the nucleus of each cell. We might call it biologically planned obsolescence. Within an individual's genes is a scheduled period of growth or development—a more or less static time of adulthood, and then a functional and structural decline. The incredibly complex act of birth, beginning with a fertilized egg and ending nine months later with a breathing, hollering little human being, is the result of a genetic plan within DNA. During the years following birth, our genetic clock ticks away, scheduling growth in spurts of development. Growth, development, and aging are not steadily unraveling, always recognizable, smooth, or regular. Children and teenagers have definite periods of rapid growth and periods of slow growth. Some young girls at the age of ten or twelve suddenly, and with little warning, are tall and busty within a few months. There are boys who develop psychological problems, difficult to outgrow, because they keep their childish figures, looks, and heights until they are 18 or 20. There are periods when children outgrow their clothes at almost breathless speeds.

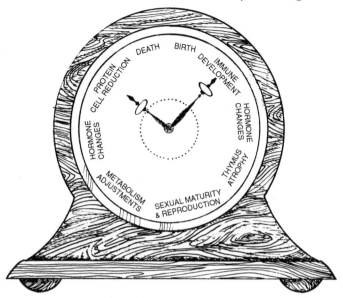

Figure 4 Genetic clock: A well-known theory of aging says that the minutes, days, and years of our lives tick away to the beat of an internal (infernal?) clock containing our life's plan.

The physical and emotional changes of aging also come about in spurts, rather than in a steady rate. One is shocked to see a few gray hairs one day in the mirror but then a year to two or three may pass with little change at all. Then one day, a further shock: Overnight the gray somehow multiplied itself. A man who is becoming bald usually notices periods when his hairbrush is relatively free of loose hair. He smiles wishfully, telling himself the fallout is finished. At other periods, he's startled to see how much of his hair collects in the brush.

The Pacific salmon shows us perhaps the most vivid example of a genetic clock at work. This amazing species of fish spawns in fresh water and the young salmon swim downstream to inhabit the ocean. In a few years, something tells them to fight their way back up the rocky rivers, rushing in a heroic display of determination and physical strength. When they reach their birthplace, they lay and fertilize eggs. And then, their biological evolutionary purpose achieved, they die. Their genetic clock sounds the alarm that affects the mechanism of the salmon's immune system. It ceases to function precisely after they have passed on their genes to the fertilized eggs and so they succumb, defenseless against infection.

There are other manifestations of the scheduled biological plan. The salmon's steroid hormone levels shoot sky-high when it is time for them to journey up the rivers, rather like an athlete's rush of adrenalin when he sees the finish line. Once their eggs are laid and fertilized, the rate of aging accelerates and the salmon in minutes take on physical aspects of old fish—a graying of the gills. They are not only the best example in biology of genetically planned aging occurring at a particular time, but also a provocative example of the possibility of our learning to adjust biological aging. Perhaps the most amazing fact about the Pacific salmon is that its biological timetable can be manipulated. By keeping the fish out at sea, by not allowing the rush upriver to take place, researchers have found that the steroid hormone rush fails to occur and the fish lives longer than it does if it climbs waterfalls and then spawns.

Another example of genetic programming occurs in the male marsupial mouse in Australia which dies at a specific time in his reproductive cycle. He exerts such aggressive energy in copulating with a female mouse that soon afterward he keels over and dies. Hormonal studies have shown the same phenomenon happening in the mouse and in the Pacific salmon—the levels of steroid hormones go up for the act of copulation and afterward the mouse's immune system shuts down so that he succumbs to infectious disease. Again, it is a genetically-controlled event that accelerates aging and death of the animal.

Accelerated aging occurs in human beings as well, although hormonal changes in people are not as well documented as in animals. The rare disease, progeria, is genetically caused. It usually kills people at about 12 years of age. Children with progeria have some of the physical characteristics of old people such as wrinkled, inelastic skin and thinning hair. Symptoms are usually not noticed until progeria babies are about a year old. Another human example of accelerated aging is Werner's syndrome, in which case the symptoms are gray hair at age 20, cataracts at 30, early skin wrinkling, and loss of muscle size. The disease seems to be a hormonal malfunction and its victims usually die around age 45 with a high frequency of cancer and vascular disease. Down's syndrome also illustrates aging as a result of genetic coding, although outside causes such as radiation, chemicals and delays in fertilization are also suspected. What happens in Down's syndrome is an early degeneration of the central nervous system, mental retardation, and a significant cancer rate (often leukemia). A highly publicized finding is that Down's syndrome babies are born with greater frequency to women who become pregnant fairly late in their reproductive years (after age 35).

A more common example of genetically planned aging, one readily seen and acknowledged, is simple family history. Aging patterns differ in human beings from family to family. In some families people usually die at age 50 or 60, in other families at age 70 or 80, and in some others at age 90 or 100. Of course, environmental conditions can alter the best laid genetic plan. For example, long exposure to asbestos fibers may cause pulmonary deficiency or emphysema in someone whose ancestors have never died from respiratory failure. A diet high in fats may lead to vascular disease in a child of a family with excellent cardiovascular systems. Cultural inheritance, in the forms of health habits learned in childhood and lifestyles modified over the years, affects the rate of aging quite aside from genetics.

Scientists are learning about genetic susceptibilities by observing laboratory mice which possess a genetic code remarkably similar to our own. Mice can be bred within "strains" or families, so that after many generations, individual mice are identical or, genetically speaking, they are homozygous. That means they have identical genes on the two arms of the chromosomes. When these mice mate, brother to sister, their recessive or weak characteristics are not eliminated as they are when matched with a more dominant gene in a different mouse. Thus, the recessive characteristics are passed along the generations of a mouse strain. This is the reason we have laws forbidding incest, for incest can weaken individuals within a species. Ancient man figured out something detrimental was caused by incest and he created religious laws forbidding it—now we have scientific evidence and we know what is happening.

Some strains of mice live 12 months; others can live 36 months and by manipulating the genetic codes of these animals we can shorten or lengthen their life spans. Another observation is that the mice who live 12 months usually die from leukemia; most of those living 36 months die from liver tumor. So not only is the rate of aging different among strains but the disease susceptibilities also are different; that tells us something about our own genetic predispositions. Within our families we share a close (but a certainly not identical) chromosomal pattern, so we share genetic susceptibilities to the same diseases. To get an idea of what we're going to die from we can look at our family history. What did our grandparents die from? This is somewhat like betting in Las Vegas, of course, and there are exceptions. But generally, family members die from the same causes unless they spend their lives in radically different environments.

A cell division experiment made by Leonard Hayflick, now at the University of Florida, has been interpreted as a good argument for the existence of a genetic clock and for the theory of genetically programmed aging. Hayflick counted the number of times that cells will divide to form daughter cells, and he found a point at which the divisions are exhausted, which is called the Hayflick limit. In a laboratory cell division can be measured because of the property some cells have which is called "contact inhibition." When they are placed in the correct medium in a dish, they will double until they completely cover the surface of the dish and then they will stop dividing. When half of them are removed exposing uncovered areas of the dish, the remaining cells will multiply again until they cover the dish a second time. This can be repeated until the capacity to divide ceases and the number of doublings can be counted.

Hayflick used a small piece of skin from a human embryo and found the cells divide fifty times, plus or minus a few doublings. When he used a piece of skin from an adult, though, there were only about twenty doublings. The cells from a child who had progeria likewise had a small number of doublings. Hayflick's interpretation is that the cells know they have a finite number of times they can divide. Is this the genetic clock?

Even if you freeze the cells, putting them in a state of suspended animation, they will resume their doublings upon thawing. Amazingly, not only do they resume, but they remember how many times they divided prior to freezing. They remember the point where they were and they finish out their remaining doublings.

When cells are frozen, (a fragile procedure), an antifreeze is necessary to keep ice crystals from forming because ice crystals puncture cells and kill them. The antifreeze chemical that is used is dimethylsulfoxide (DMSO), a drug used by many people to treat arthritis although there's no good scientific evidence that it can help. DMSO is also used in livestock breeding. A tiny calf embryo can be frozen with DMSO and later implanted in a cow at the right time for her. DMSO is potentially useful for the preservation of blood for use in emergencies and perhaps one day DMSO will open the door for cryogenics—freezing a human body indefinitely without death. Such technology does not exist yet. It is one thing to freeze a few tiny cells (which are smaller than a pinpoint) so rapidly with very cold liquid nitrogen that ice crystals will not form. It is quite another thing to immerse an adult human body with that kind of speed. Those people in the late 1960's who were frozen and are mysteriously hidden away someplace are not going to make it.

Wear and Tear and Evolution

Hayflick's interpretation of the cells' doubling capacity is that this is a good beginning point for studying aging. Other scientists are not so sure. For one thing, the Hayflick limit of cell division was determined in a laboratory, *in vitro*, and no one can say with surety that human cells cease dividing *in vivo* after fifty doublings. Those who challenge the genetic theory point to external hazards, such as ultraviolet rays from the sun, which damage or destroy our cells. Aging, they say, is the result of wear and tear on our bodies, an accumulation of inevitable errors and mutations in the genetic code. Our environment is responsible: Disease, physical injury, toxic chemicals, smog, cigarettes, free radicals—all take their toll as we go through life. These environmentally-caused mutations in the genetic code are then responsible for mistakes in the DNA-RNA processes of replication and translation, leading to our production of faulty proteins. Faulty proteins can lead to a host of breakdowns in the body: Hair loses its strength, muscle can lose fiber, nerve cells lose the power to transmit impulses from the brain to the muscles, and the immune system loses its ability to fight off infection. These malfunctions in protein production have a true domino effect, a breakdown in one area leading to further breakdowns in other areas, eventually affecting the functioning of the body's renewal capabilities.

It is often argued that wear and tear in the forms of disease and injury do not cause aging *per se*, but it cannot be denied that accumulated injuries and illnesses create a susceptibility to bad health. Chronic infection strains the defense and healing capacities of the body.

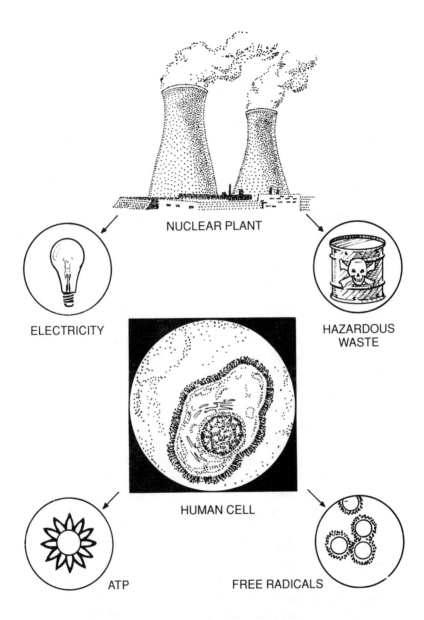

Figure 5 Pleiotropic effects: Just as the generation of nuclear energy creates harmful waste products, so the production of ATP by glucose and oxygen in the cells, throws off potentially harmful free radicals.

Besides the wear and tear argument, further doubt is placed on the cell doubling study of aging by another theory known as stem cell depletion. Stem cells are the specific cells that divide to form daughter cells. Tissue from an embryo which was used in the cell doubling experiment has potentially many more stem cells than does tissue taken from an adult. Hayflick found more than twice as many doublings in the embryo cells than in adult cells. Stem cells, however, do not differentiate and are by no means the only kind of cells we have. Their function is to reproduce exactly, not to form different cells with new functions, such as white blood cells. It is believed we have a finite number of stem cells at birth. When we lose them to environmental hazards like sunlight and physical injury, unfortunately, we don't replace them.

The evolutionary theory of aging is really a combination of the genetic and the environmental theories, but it goes further than either of the two. According to this theory, there is indeed a genetic program and it does not act alone; it is influenced by our particular environment. Environmental conditions (or challenges, as biologists like to call them) may speed up the genetic clock or, in the happy case in which good health habits, nutrition, and regular exercise constitute a body's "environment," may even slow its ineluctable ticking. The evolution of our complex bodies is due to chemical changes or mutations within molecules as a result of DNA's meeting the challenges presented by the environment. Evolution, accepted now by most scientists as fact rather than theory, explains how life was created and how it has continued on our planet. When life began, the earth's environment was nothing like what it is now—it was mostly nitrogen and methane gas, carbon dioxide, and a little oxygen. There was no layer of ozone above the earth, so most ultraviolet light from the sun came through the atmosphere, and there was an enormous amount of volcanic and electrical activity. All these constituents formed the building blocks of life as we know it; amino acids, proteins, nucleotides. Enthusiasts can mix the same constituents in a laboratory, in a Bell jar, and if they wait about a billion years they will see life forming.

At the same time that life was beginning on earth, destructive chemical processes developed as well, competing with the life-forming chemistry. These destructive processes in biology are described by the term biosenescence. Fortunately for us, when life was struggling to start, the life building processes proved to dominate in the competition with the life destroying forces.

This competitive evolutionary process of building things up and tearing things down is still with us and may be the force behind aging. Our life-building chemistry has "pleiotropic" effects, which means that two things result from the same process and sometimes, one result is good for us and the other is detrimental. An illustration is the body's conversion of energy. Inside the cell, the bacteria-like organelle called mitochondria burn sugar which generates usable energy but throws off free radicals of superoxide, a very unstable form of oxygen. It just happens; it's a part of the process. It's analogous to the production of waste products in our nuclear generating plants where the problem is that we don't know what to do with the wastes we produce. On the other hand, our bodies have come up with a way to deal with the superoxide and maybe, one day, we'll figure out how to make nuclear power safe. In our bodies we create the enzyme superoxide dismutase (SOD) which has been discussed in another context. SOD is a life-building chemical that destroys free radicals of superoxide, and our genetic plan may well call for an abundance of SOD early in our lives. Later, the amount we produce may drop considerably (again, part of the plan), allowing superoxide to accumulate and cause molecular damage. Our digestive enzymes may have a clock too, instructing them to be more abundant when we are growing and later to decrease in amount. An implication of the decrease is that we don't get as much nutritional value from food as we age since digestion and absorption are slightly slowed.

The evolutionary theory of aging says that early in our body's development, the life building processes are very much more active than the tearing-down processes. Then, at about the time of our maturity, the competitive life and anti-life forces roughly equalize. As we get older though, the genetic program slows down the life-building processes with the result that the anti-life processes begin to predominate. Some decline in the body's metabolism is inevitable. Personal effort to maintain good health can retard, but not stop, the inevitable: Good health buttresses and assists the life building processes. Exercise, good nutrition, rest, and guarding against hazards like smoking cigarettes boosts the life-building processes in their struggle against the competition.

The evolutionary theory not only explains the mechanics of the aging process—the struggle between the life and the anti-life forces—but it also explains why life ends in death. Simply put, there could be no life without death. Why?

Genetic mutation, although given a bad press because of its capacity to cause malfunction in an individual, is essentially a positive evolutionary process. Genetic change is vital if a species is to adapt and prosper—a good mixing of the gene pool being necessary for evolution. After mixing our characteristics, after we have reproduced, we're no longer needed for the evolutionary process, so we die. If this were not so, there would be no evolution and we would not be here at all.

Tracking Down the Biological Clock

If we assume that a biological clock inexorably counts down the years within the body, acting as a mechanism for evolution, our next question is, where exactly is this clock? Does it lie at the "tissue level," say, in a particular organ like the heart or the liver? And does that mean our predisposition to aging is in that spot so we will have heart disease or liver failure? Or does the clock work in all tissues of the body—an

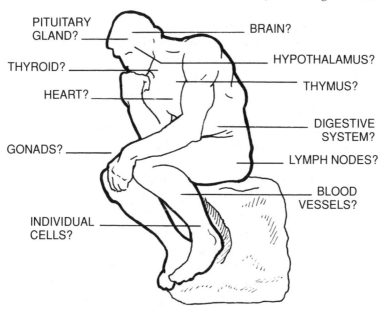

PITUITARY
GLAND?

THYROID?

HEART?

GONADS?

INDIVIDUAL
CELLS?

BRAIN?

HYPOTHALAMUS?

THYMUS?

DIGESTIVE
SYSTEM?

LYMPH NODES?

BLOOD
VESSELS?

Figure 6 Where is our genetic clock? If we accept the genetic clock theory, a puzzling challenge is to determine its location. Is it the brain? Is it hormonal? Is it the immune system?

intercellular phenomenon? Since the organs of the body interact with each other and depend on each other, perhaps the key to aging is a lack of coordination stemming from an initial problem in one area. Again, like a domino effect, functional decline in one place leads to a breakdown in a related place, and, eventually, cascades to a generalized breakdown, a sort of deregulation.

Some scant evidence for answering these questions is developing in research laboratories. Organ transplants in mice, dainty operations, have shown interesting results. If you take, for example, a young mouse's ovary and plant it in an old female mouse, it will not function very well although it was in fine shape when it was in the young mouse. What happened during the transplant? The converse shows a different result: An ovary from an old mouse placed in a young mouse won't function perfectly, but it will function better than it did when it was in the old mouse. Such experiments suggest that the state of affairs influencing an organ, the area around it, affects its ability to do its job.

Kidney transplants have extended the lives of mice by several months, with implications for our own aging. It is important to remember, however, that these experiments are done with animals which are genetically identical. Therefore the experiments are not skewed by graft rejection—the transplanted tissue is accepted as if it were the animal's own tissue. In people, however, the fact that we're not genetically identical means transplanted organs run up against the problem of tissue rejection. The problem is not the age of the tissue or the age of the donor or of the recipient; the transplant is rejected by the immune system because it is "foreign"—genetically different tissue. And another thing to consider in aging studies is that tissue is damaged by the transplant operation itself. Bone marrow grafting shows this. When old animal marrow is put into a young animal it has been found there's basically no difference in the marrow, but the wear and tear of the transplant creates scarring problems.

The cell implant work of Beatrice Mintz of the Fox Chase Cancer Institute may prove significant in our understanding of cancer, aging's most feared disease. Using a microneedle, she has placed a cancerous cell into a developing mouse embryo, keeping track of the cell by its pigment differences from the normal cells. She saw that the cancerous cell incorporated itself and formed not more cancerous cells but healthy, normal, cells. The interpretation of her experiment is that something in the cell's original environment was causing the malfunction and by putting it in a healthy environment it corrected itself. The experiment provides the hope that someday cancerous cells may be manipulated to function normally. Other scientists have grafted skin cells from aging rats to young rats and have found that such cells survived longer as part of a young host than the remaining skin left on the older animals.

Theories . . . and theories . . . and theories . . .

Trying to explain aging has generated many other theories—
so many, in fact, that it is sometimes said there are as many
theories of aging as there are gerontologists. One is the theory
of declining energy, which states all living beings have a fixed
amount of vigor and, once used, it is gone, much like a tank
of gasoline in an automobile. Adherents of this theory point
out that older people lose muscular and skeletal strength,
their cardiopulmonary systems decline in capacity, and their
ability to cope with emotional stress is compromised. Such
aging changes, however, cannot be said to affect all older
people at the same or even at similar rates. Indeed, as other
chapters in this book discuss, the loss of vitality described in
the declining energy theory is the result of bad health, not of
aging. Individuals age at different rates and there is abundant
evidence that good health habits maintained throughout
life—foremost among them regular exercise and a nutritional
diet—can revitalize energy and vigor as we age.

The collagen theory describes the general stiffening of
connective tissue that occurs in the skin, tendons, blood
vessels, and most of the body's organs. Most scientists believe
that this stiffening which is the result of the cross-linking of
molecules that impede cellular function is not the cause, but,
rather, a result of aging.

Three lesser theories describing molecular change
rightly belong under the greater heading of the genetic theory.
One, the mutation argument for aging, states that faulty cells
proliferate in the body, functional faults the inevitable result.
Over time, point mutations can strain DNA's repair mechanisms and errors in protein synthesis cascade toward an
"error catastrophe." A theory with the glamorous appellation,
garbage accumulation, holds that aging cells falter in their
function because of a build-up of waste products such as
lipofuscin that crowds out normal cellular machinery. The
free radical theory says that we age as a result of collisions

between by-products of oxidation and other molecules—events that probably cause lipofuscin wastes and molecular crosslinking.

The immune theory of aging gains more proponents as researchers steadily learn more about the body's complex defense system. Elderly people's immune response is compromised in at least two ways: initial defense against infection is slowed and their defense often turns on the body itself by what is known as autoimmunity. In several experiments, scientists have kept fish and fruit flies alive longer than normal by subjecting them to cold temperatures. It appears that coldness deters the immune response, protection against autoimmunity.

Donner Denckla and Caleb Finch, prominent among gerontologists, claim that hormones are directly involved in our aging. According to Finch, the author of many books and articles on various aspects of aging, the control of the body's biological clock lies in the neuroendocrine system. Denckla has proposed that the pituitary gland releases an aging hormone at puberty—a hormone as yet unnamed—which hinders the metabolic rate of both the cardiovascular and the immune systems. He has found that by removing the pituitary gland from laboratory rats, their circulatory and defense functions actually maintained regulation longer than expected for their species. What's more, the rats' fur renewal improved.

Hormones are our bodies' movers and shapers—our great organizers—influencing not only our physical well-being, but our intellect as well. They oversee extraordinary changes in our bodies as we develop and age. Surprisingly, the levels of many hormones remain constant throughout our lives.

Chapter 4

Hormones: Our Great Regulators

If the hormones of our bodies were perfectly known and understood—all their functions and why and when they function—diagnosing a person's physical and emotional conditions would be a simple matter of a blood test. Such a blood test doesn't exist . . . yet. Biomedicine is just beginning to understand what hormones are and how they work. Certainly not even all the body's hormones have been identified. Somewhat more than a hundred of them are known and each year the list gets longer.

What is known is fascinating. Some hormones regulate our rate of growth, development, and aging. Others lie waiting for a signal from the brain and then instantly course throughout our bloodstream, giving us a stamina boost just when we need it or providing our response to stress. At puberty, other hormones go all out, directing amazing changes in our appearance and in our emotions. After then, some new hormones come into our lives, directing the way we react to sexual stimulation and making it possible for us to conceive and to reproduce ourselves. Hormones play a role in our retention or elimination of salt; they regulate our water content, and thus, our blood pressure. After we eat something salty, hormones tell us we're thirsty. They help us to maintain a balance of the essential minerals. Two well-known hormones, insulin and glucagon, work together to regulate the amount of sugar in our blood. Gastrointestinal hormones stimulate the production of digestive enzymes in the stomach and other organs so our nutrients can be absorbed. And the endorphins, which have only recently been discovered, seem to act within the brain as natural anesthetics, helping us tolerate pain.

Hormones are our great regulators and they might be called chemical communicators. They carry messages from one place in the body to another, keeping every place aware of what is going on elsewhere. It is said that without hormones, the eye would not know what the toe is up to. When an egg is fertilized, it is a hormone that signals the mother's brain, telling it what has happened below. Then the brain instructs other hormones to stop the menstrual cycle until the baby is born. Without this series of signals, the fertilized egg would be aborted.

When our brain senses stress, a hormone with a disarming but descriptive name, adrenalcorticotrophic hormone (ACTH), is sent from the pituitary gland to the adrenal gland, and, in turn, causes another hormone, cortisol, to circulate quickly, helping us cope. This beautiful example of teamwork constitutes hormonal control. Rarely indeed, does one hormone act alone. An increase in the amount of one, like cortisol (the stress hormone) can lead to the decrease of others—the sex hormones, for example. Three of them, antidiuretic hormone, renin, and aldosterone, team up to control our blood pressure. High blood pressure or hypertension, strictly speaking, is not nervousness; it is too much pressure on the blood vessel walls—the vessels' failure to accommodate blood flow. If a blood vessel does not have the capacity to expand in times of accelerated blood flow and increased pressure, if it does not receive the hormonal message, serious cardiovascular problems can develop.

Hormones direct the momentous event we call menopause, a physical change many people think of as a benchmark—youth behind and old age ahead. Because of their role in menopause, we ageistically accused hormones, until recently, of failing us and opening the way for an acceleration of aging. Indeed, the medical treatment called hormone replacement is touted by many scientists, physicians, and post-menopausal women as a sort of fountain of youth. Other scientists are learning, however, that although hormone therapy has valuable uses, such as the retarding of aging bone and muscle loss, it won't keep us from aging and it can even have harmful effects. Although our sex hormones decrease as we age, the levels of many hormones don't fall at all. It appears, rather, that with age, hormones more typically are prevented from acting out their functions. Other changes in the body, cells, organs, and bloodstream inhibit hormonal regulation. Growth hormone, most active when we're babies and young children, changes in function after we're grown and decreases very slightly if at all. It continues to stimulate our adult replacement of cells and tissues.

The pituitary gland, influenced by the hypothalamus, sends thyroid stimulating hormone (TSH), a "releasing factor," to the thyroid gland, providing the signal for the release of thyroxin, which maintains the body's metabolic rate. It acts to increase the oxygen consumption in almost all our bodily tissues. Besides growth, development, and maintenance, it is known to influence nervous system activity and has a regulatory role in our utilization of fats and carbohydrates. A recent study published in The Journal of Gerontology found that the somatomedins, a group of insulin-like hormones, decrease with age. In men aged 58 to 80, researchers found one-third less of these hormones than in men aged 23 to 27. The somatomedins help us to make cartilage, bone, and muscle, so evidence of their decreasing levels represents an important step in explaining musculoskeletal disorders in some elderly people. Another study points to obesity as a cause of decreased levels of growth hormone. This research provided evidence that obese people have a pituitary defect resulting in an impairment of the releasing factor sent to the thyroid. What's more, the levels of another hormone, somatostatin, which inhibits the release of growth hormone, was found to increase in obese people. There is evidence, moreover, that the situation can be corrected with weight loss.

From Zsa Zsa Gabor to King Kong

Each of us, whether we are male or female, has a mixture of male and female sex hormones. When we are developing in our mother's uterus, we are exposed to her particular mixture of hormones and to her particular hormonal cycles. Our sexual characteristics are set at this early stage of development. But you cannot look at a just-born baby and know that in twenty years he will look like King Kong, if a male, or if a female, that she will turn out with the exact femininity of Zsa Zsa Gabor. Each person, male or female, will develop sexual characteristics uniquely his or her own, and will develop them at puberty because of sex hormones whose levels were set during the uterine stage of development. A person's physical characteristics can range from ultra-feminine to super-macho, dainty and smooth-skinned to swarthy and lumbering, with an abundance of unwanted (or highly prized) hair. There are many shades of gray from King Kong to Zsa Zsa Gabor.

In the past, it has been said that hormones are responsible for homosexuality. Scientists and psychologists, however, don't believe that today. Although it is true that certain rare diseases like testicular feminization can occur, they now believe that sexual orientation is learned. Testicular feminization is a genetic or inborn error resulting in the body's failure to respond to the male hormone, testosterone, and female sex characteristics develop in a male body. It is very possible that an individual unfortunate enough to have this disease could grow up assuming he's female even though his chromosomes are male. (People with this disease are sterile.) But sexual preference such as homosexuality seems to be determined by environment and learning, not by hormones.

The decrease in sex hormones that occur as we age is a good argument for both the genetic and the evolutionary theories of aging. The sex hormones function primarily so that we will reproduce, continuing to evolve our species. And they stimulate us to do just that during the years of our lives when we're healthiest and at our peak physically. After we're past that period, the sex hormones are apparently programmed to wane. At puberty, the hypothalamus in the brain signals the beginning of our sex cycle, sending hormones to the nearby pituitary gland, which, in turn, sends out hormones that circulate in the bloodstream, causing still more hormonal secretions when they reach the sex organs. In women, the ovary secretes estrogen; in men, the testes secrete testosterone. In women the level of estrogen climaxes monthly with the release of an egg from the ovary; in men the testosterone level comes and goes in waves, but continues daily. Why this difference? We hardly need science to explain what is obvious: carrying and nurturing a child is manifestly more complex than the male role of merely participating in fertilization.

When an egg is fertilized, a steroid hormone, progesterone, is stimulated and carries the message to the hypothalamus that it is time to stop the cycle of sex hormones. Thus, progesterone is called the pregnancy hormone; it stops the menstrual flow which would otherwise abort the egg from the uterus. A synthetic form of progesterone, diethylstilbestrol (DES) given to women beginning in the late nineteen-forties if their pregnancies appeared to be naturally aborting, proved more potent than expected. DES assisted in bringing the pregnancies to term, mimicking the action of progesterone, but years later some of the children developed cancer or had an increased risk of cancer. About one of every thousand DES daughters has had cervical cancer at a young age—between 14 and 25 years old. As the reports of these occurrences came to light, the use of DES halted. It was not an easily learned lesson in the unpredictable side effects of steroid hormones.

DES has left other legacies. Many of the daughters, about twenty percent of them, have incurred pregnancy problems of their own, such as premature birth. Among the DES sons, there have been reports of abnormal sperm and, also, maldescent of the testes (a known risk of testicular cancer, although none of the young men have so far actually reported cancerous growth). The most recent revelation of the after effects of DES is breast cancer in some of the women who used the synthetic hormones. One study of six thousand women who were given DES in pregnancy found a significantly higher rate of breast cancer than would be present in the normal population. Their lumps developed twenty to thirty years after pregnancy. Many physicians now advise women who used DES to give themselves monthly breast self-examinations, take an annual medical exam, and, if they're past 50, to have an annual mammogram.

The history of the use of DES is indeed shocking but the footnote is obscene: Much of the research which might have yielded more knowledge (leading to preventive treatment for maladies yet unknown) has been shelved by the federal budget cuts of the early 1980s.

Synthetic forms of estrogen and progesterone are used today with supposed safety in birth control pills which send a false signal of pregnancy to the brain. The body is chemically fooled into thinking it is pregnant and thus, the normal hormones which cause release of an egg do not get sent to the ovary. The pills can prevent a fertilized egg's implantation on the inner walls of the uterus so, in essence, an abortion has been caused, and that is the scientific basis for religious opposition to this form of birth control.

Carrying the Messages

How do hormones do their jobs? When we need a shot of adrenalin (or epinephrine, as adrenalin is now called) how does the brain relay its instruction to the adrenal gland that the hormones must be secreted? When the ovary readies an egg for fertilization, it is responding to a particular hormone that came from the pituitary gland with the express purpose of stimulating an egg. Why does that particular hormone go to the ovary and not to, say, the lungs or heart?

Through the bloodstream a hormone goes everywhere. It circulates throughout our bodies along with oxygen, nutrients, and proteins. It happens that a hormone is equipped with a mechanism that tells it when it has reached its "target organ;" a hormone whose target is the ovary travels to other organs besides the ovary but it will not stimulate any activity anywhere except in the ovary. It knows to pass through those other places and then stop when it arrives at the ovary. The mechanism is performed by molecules called receptors.

Hormones and the cells of their targets are equipped with these molecular structures and fit each other like pieces of a jigsaw puzzle. When a hormone fits the receptors in the cells of an organ, it knows it has found its target and it stays there; that is where it is supposed to be. Scientists describe this attraction of receptors and their hormones as "molecular binding." It is Mother Nature's ingenious way of joining molecules—on a temporary basis. We and all other forms of life have evolved because of the binding and therefore the building of basic organic compounds.

There are several types of hormones and their differences are mainly those of function. Although they work in different ways, they are all hormones because they are chemical communicators—they pass messages along for the purpose of regulating the whole body. One type, the polypeptides, have an amino acid-chain structure like the proteins made from the genetic code in RNA. Insulin is a polypeptide hormone, but unlike insulin, which comes from the pancreas, most polypeptide hormones come from the pituitary gland just below the brain. Polypeptides are usually sent to endocrine glands, their targets, like the thyroid gland or the

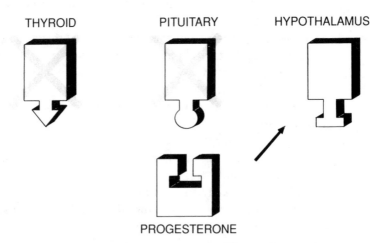

THYROID   PITUITARY   HYPOTHALAMUS

PROGESTERONE

Figure 7   Molecular binding: Hormones find their "target organs" because their molecules contain receptors which fit their target like pieces of a jigsaw puzzle. In the example shown here, progesterone locks onto the hypothalamus because the receptor and target match, and not onto the thyroid or pituitary because they do not.

adrenal gland, to stimulate secretion of other hormones. They bind to receptors that are integral parts of the target cells' membranes.

Steroid hormones, notably stress and sex hormones, differ from polypeptides in their structure. They pass right through the membranes of cells where, on the inside, free-floating receptors lie waiting and will bind to them. Cholesterol in our bodies makes our steroid hormones. If we don't get an adequate supply of cholesterol-producing nutrients in our diet, enzymes go into action to make it for us. Vitamin A is now believed to be a hormone stored and secreted by the liver. It has characteristics of a steroid hormone and one place in which it functions is the retina. Forms of Vitamin A help to capture photons of light in the process of vision. Vitamin D, also a steroid-like hormone, assists calcium in forming our bones.

Thyroid hormone works like both polypeptide hormones and steroids, acting on the surfaces of cells as well as inside them. Besides its primary job of overseeing how we use nutrients and oxygen, it regulates our basic metabolism, our production of heat for the energy that keeps us going. A deficiency of iodine, a part of thyroid hormone, can cause a goiter (a large lump in the throat). Since the advent of iodized salt in our diet, however, goiter is now very rare.

The other two types of hormones are neurotransmitters and prostaglandins. Not everyone agrees about labelling them as hormones, but they meet the definition: they are chemical communicators. Neurotransmitters sometimes enter the bloodstream, but they normally travel the lengths of nerve cells. When they reach the end of the line (the edge of a nerve cell), they leap through open space to another nearby nerve cell, in the process, carrying electrical impulses from one nerve to another. The prostaglandins were discovered originally in the prostate gland (which explains their name). It is not yet known how they work, but they somehow initiate our defense whenever an injury occurs somewhere on or in the body. It appears they function as a sort of burglar alarm, rushing from the point of injury to alert the immune system that there is a job to be done. They also play a role in ovulation and help to stimulate contractions of the uterus during labor.

Because several hormones generally act together in an "axis," one stimulating another in a cycle, it is very difficult to pinpoint their relation to our aging changes. One must look at all the different points of activity in an axis to find where a change begins, affecting the subsequent hormones in the cycle. In the case of the thyroid gland, its hormones are first triggered by trophic hormones from the pituitary, which have specific target organs. The levels of these thyroid hormones in the bloodstream tell the pituitary that more or less is needed. When there is a change in the thyroid hormones, we must ask: Is it in one of the target organs? The answer is that it could be in any of these places.

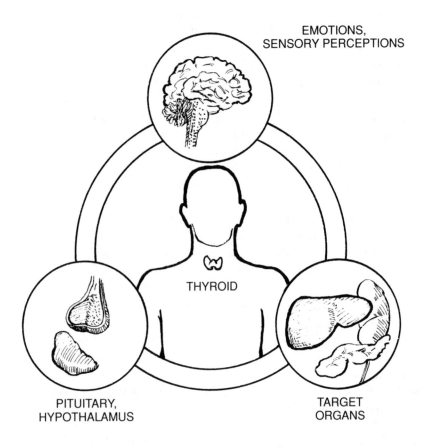

EMOTIONS,
SENSORY PERCEPTIONS

THYROID

PITUITARY,
HYPOTHALAMUS

TARGET
ORGANS

Figure 8 Why do hormone levels change with age? This illustration highlights several influences on the thyroid gland which may cause changes in the levels of hormones it releases. Not only does the gland itself change, it may react to sensory and emotional signals from the brain, changes in quantities of releasing hormones from the hypothalamus and pituitary, or changes in size and number of its "target" organs. Changes in blood flow and in levels of circulating hormones also may affect the thyroid.

But this is not all. The hypothalamus in the brain also sends releasing hormones to the nearby pituitary gland. They tell the pituitary to send its hormones to the thyroid. So the functioning of the pituitary-thyroid axis can be chemically regulated or it can be started and stopped by the brain. And the brain, it must be remembered, is responding to our sensory perception. Thus, hormonal control is affected by what we think, what we sense, and what we feel. Changes as we age can therefore be related to problems at many places— the pituitary, the thyroid, the target organs (which may not be so receptive to hormones as they used to be), or the brain. And yet a further complication. One must not forget that age-onset changes in circulation will obviously affect the secretion and the transportation of hormones.

Most evidence from scientific studies appears to show that thyroid hormone levels do not decrease with age, but rather, their target organs may malfunction and therefore fail to utilize the thyroid hormones. There is also evidence that the quantity of receptors for many hormones decrease as we age. So, although a hormone is flowing at its normal level, less of it actually binds to its target. Some evidence shows that the stimulating signals from the hypothalamus are lessened with aging, implicating the brain as the primary source of change.

Hormones and Sex Drive

Changes in sex hormones as we age are understood a little better although the specific physical starting point of menopause is still not known. The cycle of sex hormones is called the ovary-pituitary axis in women, or the testes-pituitary axis in men. The pituitary gland sends stimulating hormones to the ovary or testes, which then release estrogen in women, testosterone in men. High or low levels of these two hormones in the bloodstream tell the pituitary that more or less is needed. The hypothalamus, again, is a factor. Our feelings are translated through the hypothalamus which triggers the pituitary. Thus, stress, desire, fatigue, and our emotions all influence the levels of our sex hormones.

Estrogen and testosterone quantities definitely decline with age. In men, the decline is gradual and may be hardly noticeable. Women, on the other hand, can't fail to notice— although menopause is rarely an abrupt change. Generally, a woman's menstrual cycles will gradually become irregular in her late forties or early fifties, much like the irregularity she knew at puberty when the cycles began in the first place. The release of estrogen from the ovary falls markedly by the time menopause is over and this, in turn, causes an increase in the release of pituitary hormones. Menopausal symptoms vary in degree from woman to woman: vaginitis, (dryness, sometimes with bleeding), heat flushes (sometimes showing a patchy redness), a thinning of the skin (especially on the face and hands), loss of breast size, and loss of bone formation. Sex drive and sexual enjoyment for many post-menopausal women increases, though, since the fear of pregnancy is gone.

The lower level of testosterone in aging men corresponds to a decreased amount of sperm made in the testes. But it is not clear whether this sperm count reduction is hormonally related or if it is due to aging blood vessels in the testes. At any rate, sex drive in men is not dependent on sperm production; sex drive is psychological for the most part.

Is menopause caused by a failure of the ovary to produce estrogen? Or is it the result of a malfunction either in the hypothalamus or the pituitary, causing over-stimulation of the ovary? Scientists generally believe that the ovary is where menopause is programmed to begin and this may be related to the number of eggs carried in the ovary. A very young girl has hundreds of thousands; the menopausal woman has only about ten thousand. On the other hand, there are the animal experiments referred to in the last chapter which show that transplants of "old" ovaries into young females result in normal ovarian cycling. Those results have led to a belief that the failure must be, somehow, in the area or "environment" of the ovary. On still another hand, some other experiments have shown that aging mice have fewer receptor cells for the binding of estrogen in the hypothalamus portion of the brain. Perhaps menopause starts in the brain.

Hormone Replacement

Many women have been relieved of menopausal depression and heat flushes by taking estrogen in one or more of several different forms. Creams containing estrogen can be effective preventives for mild vaginitis, but no one advocates such treatment for all women. Simply put, the facts about estrogen replacement are not all in yet. Some clear dangers are well known: High doses of estrogen can lead to endometrial cancer, cardiopulmonary problems such as hypertension and thromboembolic disease, and diabetes can be aggravated. Administration of estrogen by "dermal patch," it is believed, makes for less risk than oral administration. Also, some studies have suggested that small doses of progestin, taken along with estrogen, can prevent endometrial cancer. The truth, however, is that the effects of progestin are not yet known either.

For men, testosterone replacement risks creating prostate gland disorders. And it is well known that most hormones, in excessive amounts, can cause liver problems. Since hormones work in concert, one affecting another, an imbalance of one leads to improper regulation of others. In replacement therapy, this fact must be considered.

Osteoporosis

Estrogen (or testosterone) replacement is felt to have a "favorable benefit-risk ratio" for persons who suffer from postmenopausal bone loss, but it only occasionally helps for

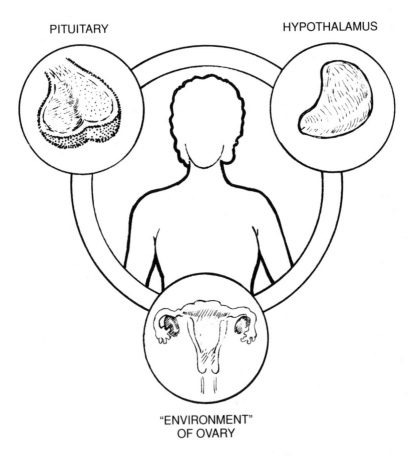

PITUITARY HYPOTHALAMUS

"ENVIRONMENT"
OF OVARY

Figure 9 What sets menopause in motion? Does menopause get underway because of changes in the hypothalamus?
Does the hypothalamus, around age 45, have fewer receptors
for hormones to trigger ovulation? Or is the menstrual pattern
changed because of a pituitary malfunction? Does the process, conversely, begin in the "environment" of the ovary
itself by, say, a reduced number of egg cells or a lower level of
estrogen?

more than five or ten years in retarding osteoporosis (an aging bone disorder that occurs in both sexes, but is far more prevalent in women). About one-third of all Caucasian women have decreased bone formation by their mid-sixties. Oriental women and black women have less of a bone mass decrease as they age, but, except for genetic differences among the races, the reasons are unknown. Nor is it known why obese Caucasian women maintain more of their bone tissue mass than thin women, but they do.

With osteoporosis, the bones become thin and more brittle—especially those bones in the pelvis and limbs. Normally, the material in human bones is never static but is always being remodeled. What happens in osteoporosis is that new bone mass is not made at the same rate it is lost and, in particular, there is more loss of trabecular bone (the connective crossbars of tissue that holds bones together) than there is loss of compact bone. Besides this age-related loss of bone, menopause is believed to be a factor in the onset of osteoporosis, as well as the failure to develop sufficient bone mass as a young adult, an increased aging sensitivity to parathyroid hormone, and malabsorption of calcium in the gastrointestinal tract.

Most people with osteoporosis suffer aches and pains, especially in the back. "Crush fractures" are common as the vertebral joints give way and compress. The pulpy nuclei of the vertebral discs lose mass too, due to a small but generalized dehydration in our bodies as we age. Along with crush fractures this can mean shrinkage in body height. Some women develop dorsal kyphosis or "dowager's hump," as a weakened spinal column gives way to a pulling forward above the waist. Osteoporosis is also responsible for more serious bone fractures, most commonly of the hip and wrist. Hip fractures in elderly women can be grave situations since the complications arising from being bedridden often lead to death.

Osteoporosis in many cases can be prevented or its effects can be lessened by diet and exercise. Adult bones and muscles need calcium—a fact that has not been stressed in the past. Some physicians recommend at least two glasses of milk a day, plus vitamin D supplementation. Calcium is also available in green vegetables. Soft drinks should be avoided by women prone to osteoporosis because they contain phosphates, something the diet needs but only in a proper balance with calcium. Too often, the phosphate-calcium balance in the contemporary diet is one-sided because of our affinity for soft drinks.

The bones need exercise just as they need calcium. Medical reports from American and Russian space flights have shown that astronauts develop osteoporosis because they are inactive; that is, their jobs consist of sedentary work since it is performed in a gravity free environment with no resistance to muscular effort. Periodontal disease (the loss of bone around the roots of the teeth) is often an early sign of osteoporosis. Chewing on bones, carrots, or crusty bread is good exercise for the teeth and, along with regular brushing and flossing, can prevent bone resorption. Cigarette smoking, alcohol, cortisol, and diabetes are all factors which can aggravate bone loss.

Safe treatment of osteoporosis includes analgesics for back pain, hyperextension exercises to strengthen the back muscles, milk, and vitamin A supplements. Oral calcium supplements and sex hormones are also used but they can cause problems. Calcium supplementation taken for long periods of time may produce, ironically, secondary decreases in bone formation. Some doctors treat bone loss with synthetic anabolic hormones such as oxandrolone, but their effects can sometimes be virilization. Sodium fluoride and calcium is occasionally prescribed in a regimen, but, as with progestin, the long-term safety of such treatment is not known.

Men with osteoporosis are often given testosterone replacement every two or three weeks in a much smaller regimen than women receiving estrogen. The problem with this, too, is a potential stimulation of prostate cancer or hypertrophy.

Diabetes

Diabetes ranks third, after cardiovascular disease and cancer, among the contemporary death-dealing diseases in the United States. Why can diet and exercise help so much in diabetes? A close look at the disease shows why. In diabetes there is a failure of hormonal regulation of the amount of glucose in our bloodstream. Insulin, the hormone secreted by the beta cells in the pancreas when they sense the presence of glucose, normally triggers other cells in our bodies to utilize the glucose which we get not just from sugar, but from all carbohydrates. In the cells, the glucose is burned and turned into energy for our use. Insulin also triggers the liver to turn sugar into glycogen, our starch, and store it for future energy use; it also tells fat cells to take sugar for longterm energy storage. As do most hormones, insulin works in concert with glucagon, which should provide a balance. Glucagon and insulin regulate our blood sugar so the level doesn't fall too low—a condition called hypoglycemia, at the other extreme from hyperglycemia.

Although there is a decrease in the amount of insulin in some people as they age, the failure of glucose regulation in many diabetics seems to result not from an insulin deficiency, but rather from a failure of the body to respond to insulin. Insulin injections are not always necessary for these people; they have enough of the hormone. Their problem lies in the receptor cells for insulin because of either a decrease in the number of receptors or their failure to recognize insulin as it circulates around them. When the insulin does not do its job, for whatever reason, the sugar goes unburned, so to speak. By reducing big surges of carbohydrates in their diets; by eating a normal caloric intake but spreading it into small meals between their regular meals; and by exercising regularly to increase the energy required and, therefore, the amount of sugar burned, many diabetics can assist their hormonal regulation.

The glucose tolerance test is used for diagnosing diabetes. The ideal way to be tested is to fast ten to sixteen hours after three days of normal diet and normal activity. After the fast, oral glucose or carbohydrate is taken and the blood level of glucose is checked at thirty minute intervals for two hours. If the last blood check plus one other show elevated glucose levels, the diagnosis can be made—although it must be remembered that there are factors which can skew the test results. Many drugs are associated with impaired glucose tolerance, including diuretics, antihypertensives, analgesics, psychoactives such as lithium carbonate and haloperidol, and some neurologic agents such as levodopa. Niacin can also upset the glucose level, as can stress.

Diet and exercise are particularly important for elderly people with diabetes because it is difficult for them to receive insulin without developing hypoglycemia which often leads to a comatose condition known as insulin shock. A normal diet with attention to carbohydrate intake is most often recommended for non-obese diabetics. Those noninsulin dependent diabetics who are overweight, though, should decrease their calories and decrease the fat in their diets to reduce the risk of coronary heart disease. Fruits and artificially sweetened drinks are recommended. A list of "OK" foods which was put out by the American Diabetes Association pointedly omits fast-foods such as burgers, shakes, pizza, macaroni and cheese, and convenience foods such as condensed soups and frozen dinners.

A Medical Primer on the Types of Diabetes

Many people have some form of diabetes (there are five separate forms) and can forestall the worst effects of their disease with diet and exercise. Actually, diabetes is now thought to be a syndrome for a group of diseases that can lead to blindness, kidney failure, susceptibility to viral infections, and the thickening of blood vessels, which can result in poor blood flow and gangrenous cysts, often requiring amputation of feet and legs.

The term "diabetes mellitus" was used until recently to describe two forms of the condition, juvenile onset diabetes and maturity onset diabetes. The former became known as insulin-dependent diabetes since it is characterized by an insulin deficiency and its victims require insulin injections. It is now called Type I diabetes and it is believed that viral infections trigger its abrupt onset usually in people under age 25, and most often in fall and winter. It is a seasonal disease. Perhaps the responsible virus selects the beta cells in the exotically named Islets of Langerhans, for it is this part of the pancreas where autoimmune destruction has been observed in Type I diabetes. And it is from these particular cells that insulin is secreted in healthy pancreases. Due to this discovery, the autoimmune nature of Type I diabetes (similar to the pathogenesis of rheumatic heart disease), early detection is now possible.

The maturity onset form of the disease, called non-insulin dependent diabetes for a time, has now been named Type II diabetes, and, unlike Type I's rapid onset, its nature is insidious. By the time many people find they have the Type II syndrome, they are developing vascular disease, neuropathy, retinopathy, and kidney disease as well. Type II has two distinct forms of its own: it is different in obese and non-obese people.

There is also a form called gestational diabetes, characterized by a glucose intolerance which develops during pregnancy; a form of diabetes bearing some of the symptoms of pancreatic disease, showing changes in hormones other than insulin, sometimes resulting from the administration of certain drugs, and related to genetics and malnourishment; and a pre-diabetes condition seen in people who have an impaired glucose tolerance. The latter form is not really diabetes, but people whose plasma levels of glucose are somewhere between normal and diabetic should certainly attend to their diet.

Diabetics have a condition known as hyperglycemia, caused by uncontrolled glucose, because regulation by insulin is not up to par and excessive levels of stress hormones such as glucagon and cortisol are circulating in their systems. Symptoms to watch for include polyuria (the passing of a large volume of urine in a short period of time) thirst, hunger, weight loss, and, in men, impotence. Diabetes, like osteoporosis, can be alleviated or, in many cases, prevented by diet and exercise. Making the effort is well worth it, for diabetics have twice the risk of normal persons for atherosclerosis, the vascular disease in which plaques of cholesterol and other substances block the flow of blood through the arteries. This may cause coronary heart disease and heart attacks. Another vascular danger comes from thickened capillary membranes—especially in the legs, kidneys, and in the retina. The neurological danger for diabetics is demyelination of the nerves (the loss of the insulating sheath around neurons) with sensory, motor, and autonomic nervous system disturbances.

Stress and the Steroid Hormones

Stress, whether physical or psychological, prompts a hormonal flow in our pituitary-adrenal gland axis. The stress hormones, steroids, go into action to protect us at those moments when we need all of our resources. The emotional rigors of going through a divorce produce one sort of stress. Being hit by a car in a crosswalk is physically stressful. Being fired from a job, or being raped, or the death of a loved one, are the kinds of stressful events influencing the release of hormones.

The adrenal glands secrete stress hormones like epinephrine, aldosterone, and cortisol which generally affect the rate of metabolism by hastening the breakdown of starches and fatty acids, resulting in a rapid supply of energy needed for dealing with stress. They also direct an increased blood supply to the heart, lungs, and skeletal muscle, diverting it from the stomach and the gastrointestinal tract. When one is hit by a car or fired from a job, the last thing he feels at the moment is hunger. That is because the stress hormones are temporarily empowering him to deal with events more urgent than eating.

Cortisol is our primary stress hormone. It is the result of a message from the brain, a reaction to danger or anxiety, which triggers the polypeptide hormone from the pituitary gland (ACTH) which then goes to the adrenal gland with instructions for the secretion of cortisol. Because it is a steroid hormone, cortisol enters the cells of the body by binding to receptors. When it arrives at the nucleus of a cell, it affects the expression of the genetic code in DNA. Figuratively speaking, cortisol temporarily substitutes its emergency "coping" instructions so the body can adjust its metabolism to meet the challenge of the particular stress it is facing.

The stress hormones are indispensable in our facing the world around us, but a problem of contemporary human life is that we call upon them for assistance inordinately often. Stress is not all bad, to be sure. The daily sort of stress, such as having to meet deadlines at work or getting the kids to school on time, is beneficial to us. It helps us to do what we must do. But an abundance of stress, such as continuous family strife, monthly financial dilemmas, bumper-to-bumper traffic everytime we drive somewhere, and so on, a daily onset of stress, causes an abundance of cortisol, related hormones, and interacting hormones. Scientific research is finding out that just as in the case of the Pacific salmon whose steroid hormones turn off their immune defenses so they fall prey to infections and die, cortisol in great amounts or in more than occasional secretions causes us great harm. Many studies are being reported of lymphadenopathies and other cancers in persons who have been treated with heavy doses of steroid hormones. Animal studies show that chronic stress, the nature of which stimulates steroid hormone flow, can lead to cancer without a doubt. Steroid hormones are designed to aid us temporarily in moments when we need a buttressed defense system. But if they usurp the immune system in more than a temporary role they are quite dangerous. They are serious drugs, some of the most powerful in our ever widening drug dependency.

Chapter 5

We Are the Drug Culture

If a person drinks neither coffee nor alcohol and never smokes, he is a member of a minority group. Caffeine, alcohol, and nicotine are unquestionably our society's drugs of choice, and aspirin is not far behind. We rarely remember that these substances are drugs, but that's what they are.

Antibiotics like penicillin and tetracycline are the true "miracle drugs" of our century, along with vaccines to prevent diseases such as polio and smallpox. The invention of drugs for fighting bacterial infections and for preventing viral diseases caused us to be hopeful, in the Forties and Fifties, that we could cure practically any ailment by finding a drug (or a "magic bullet," as some redblooded American scientists and physicians put it) to shoot at it. Since then, scientists and physicians have learned that fighting disease is an infinitely more complex problem than ridding a frontier of outlaws, and they've lately transferred their hopes for eradicating disease to molecular biology. It may one day be possible through recombinant-DNA techniques to bolster our own immune system capabilities so that we resist infection altogether. Nevertheless we are, at this moment, a drug culture. Indeed, our reliance on drugs is increasing, not diminishing.

Sometimes we overdo it. We tend to believe that there is a pill for every illness. Not long ago, street-corner mountebanks promised good health from elixirs of highly-concentrated alcohol. More recently, physicians have encouraged us to think we can feel better simply by putting chemicals in our bloodstream. As a result, if the doctor doesn't give us a prescription we don't believe we've got our money's worth.

Analgesics like Darvon and antianxiety drugs such as Valium are almost staples in the daily lives of many people. The old saying, "An apple a day keeps the doctor away," now reads, "Did you take your medicine today?" (Actually, the word of choice is "medication.") It is certainly true that drugs are miraculous. They are one of the reasons we now look forward to the new human longevity. But at the same time, they can be quite dangerous. Too often they have pleiotropic effects; like oxygen and its particles known as free radicals, drugs help us in one way but can harm us in another way. Amphetamines used as diet pills may have caused addictions more often than they aided in weight loss. In some sad cases, a drug may do more than it is intended to do; it causes side effects which necessitate another drug, and another, and another. Unfortunately, this is a common situation in the sick elderly. Have they allowed themselves to become too dependent on what easily becomes a vicious circle?

Biological changes in the aging body significantly affect drug dosage and the interactions of drugs taken simultaneously. It would not be altogether accurate to say that before physicians became attuned to aging's effects on drugs, many elderly people unwittingly suffered prescription abuse. The truth is that many of them still fall victims to overreliance on drug therapy with knowledgeable multiple-drug consideration.

The story of an old man in a small coal mining area of Pennsylvania illustrates the problem. Eighty-one years old, he was fit and healthy until one afternoon when he was driving his old pickup truck down the hilly highway to Allentown to visit with his grandchildren, his favorite pastime. Out of the blue, a severe heart attack gripped him, but he had the strength of body and mind to safely pull off to the side of the road where a passerby called for help.

In the hospital, the old man was given tranquilizers and

pain relievers along with several drugs for stabilizing blood flow and heart rhythm and although his heart recovered with little lasting damage, he began to experience mental lapses. He was so confused upon leaving the hospital that he didn't even recognize his grandchildren. His behavior was so inappropriate for him that they took him back to the hospital where his condition was diagnosed as organic brain syndrome with irreversible dementia. Increasing the dosage of his tranquilizers, his doctors also recommended a nursing home for the old man.

Not accepting such a prognosis, one of the grandchildren, a young woman who happened to work as an aide in a convalescent home, took her grandfather to another physician who almost immediately declared the case to be "senility caused by medication." The new doctor gradually stopped the tranquilizers, and in a matter of weeks the 81 year old was back in his pickup truck, perfectly in touch with reality except for one lapse of memory: he had absolutely no recollection of his short stay in the nursing home.

Molecular Actions of Drugs

Drugs and hormones work in similar ways. An exogenously-supplied hormone is, in fact, a drug, in contrast to endogenous hormones, those which our bodies produce. Drugs, like hormones, usually have specific targets within the body and they, too, work by the molecular chemistry of binding. Molecules of a drug bind to receptors for which they are intended, sometimes receptors on the surface of antigens or sometimes receptors on certain cells of the body. Antibiotics have a systemic effect—when they enter the bloodstream, they travel to all parts of the body, although they will bind only to certain surfaces. If we take an antibiotic for a throat infection the drug doesn't hang only in the throat. It circulates in the blood and diffuses through cells, even to the surface of our skin where it may react with sunlight to cause a rash. That is why instructions such as staying out of sunlight accompany certain antibiotics.

How does penicillin do its job? It has a receptor seeking mechanism and it destroys bacteria since they have receptors for it. The reason it destroys bacteria without causing damage to our own cells is that we don't have these particular receptors on our cells. Bacteria are cells with DNA and ribosomes, like our cells, but, unlike human cells, they do not have a nucleus and their cell wall resembles the cellulose of plants. Bacteria have a particular enzyme which makes their cell walls and penicillin binds to this enzyme, inhibiting it from making the cell wall. Without a cell wall to encase them, the "nude" bacteria break open and since they can't make the complex carbohydrates for their coat which is necessary for their existence, they die.

Our cells have neither cell walls made of complex carbohydrates nor cell wall enzymes like those of bacteria and so penicillin does not interfere with our own cells' activities. Some people suffer an allergic reaction to penicillin because their particular genetic codes have instructed their immune systems to fight off penicillin, a foreign object which is invading them. Perhaps they were exposed to penicillin early in their development, since it is a rather ubiquitous substance which occurs, for instance, in bread mold. It can get into foodstuffs such as milk because sick cows are often treated with it. A breast-feeding baby may be exposed if his mother is being treated with penicillin. The baby doesn't notice a thing, but his immune system has seen the foreign substance and will remember it. Later, when the child is given penicillin for a sore throat, his immune system will marshal its forces and attack the drug as if it were a viral invasion. This is called an allergic reaction. It may be accompanied by physiological shock, but in actuality, an allergic reaction to penicillin is extremely rare. Perhaps one in almost four thousand people is really allergic to penicillin to the point that the situation is life-threatening. Most people who believe they cannot use the drug probably remember a sore spot from a previous injection, mere muscle or nerve damage from a badly placed needle. Therefore they believe penicillin is bad for them, that they are allergic to it, and they use alternative antibiotics that may be potentially more dangerous to them. Antibiotics are not all so benign relative to human cells as penicillin; many of them are toxic to the liver, kidneys, or other cellular tissue.

"Interfere" and "inhibit" are words that describe the ways most drugs do what they do. Interferon is a beautifully named drug, because it interferes when a virus attempts to take over a normal cell. Tetracycline interferes with the making of proteins in bacteria, their ability to stay alive, by binding to the ribosomes. Cancer drugs used in chemotherapy are called "nucleic acid synthesis inhibitors" because they bind to enzymes that make nucleic acids, an action that is not as specific as that of antibiotics. They stop not only cancerous cells from growing, but unfortunately, normal cell growth, too, for they interfere with enzymes that are making DNA. The problem with the many chemotherapy drugs is that they inhibit DNA production in all the tissues of the body, not just in the cancerous places. Cancer patients on chemotherapy become nauseated because the drugs stop cell growth and repair in the intestine. Losing hair is only one of many deleterious side effects—bone and muscle cell turnover is compromised and the immune system cannot provide proper surveillance against infection.

Acyclovir is an antiviral drug which inhibits viral replication without harm to our cells. Used for restraining severe herpes virus infections, the drug may damage the kidney when it is used simultaneously with many other drugs, and it can cause an adverse nervous system reaction with alcohol. Acyclovir is not one hundred percent effective either, as many people who have tried it have discovered with some dismay. But it is only a beginning of antiviral weapons made possible by genetic technology. Already acyclovir derivatives such as BW 759U and 6-deoxyacyclovir, in experimental use, are proving effective against the elusive cytomegalovirus and the Epstein-Barr virus.

Aging and Heightened Drug Effects

A general rule to be remembered about the relation between drugs and aging is that drugs have a heightened effect in us as we grow older. Changes in weight and height are two important adjustments we make as we age, and they affect drug dosage. Most of the body's organs adjust their functional capacity as we age, and their capacity to absorb drugs changes. A loss of up to thirty percent of our lean body mass as we age affects the retention and the elimination of drugs. Further, since drugs depend on the circulatory system to carry them through the body and to the genitourinary sites for elimination from the body, cardiovascular aging changes become important considerations in prescribed drug therapy and in our non-prescription drug consumption.

During the course of our adult years, say, from 25 to 75, we may lose as much as two inches in height. Our spines compress because our vertebral discs flatten. Vertebral discs have a pulpy, almost liquid center, and because of gradual dehydration in these centers over the years, the vertebral column compresses. As we age, we lose liquid in many of our tissues other than the bones. The interstitial spaces in our bodies (the areas between organs) are not filled with air as it would appear from anatomical models of human beings. Rather, these spaces are liquid—water, blood, and an assortment of chemicals. As dehydration occurs almost everywhere, our entire solid mass settles downward and we lose height. Osteoporosis, if we are developing it, will hasten the shrinking.

A loss of height over the years implies the necessity of eating less, drinking less, and using smaller quantities of therapeutic drugs. A smaller body mass at age 65 simply does not need the same amounts of calories that a 30-year old body requires, nor can it metabolize as quickly the same drug dosage prescribed for a young adult. This adjustment does not happen overnight; it is a gradual change taking place during the aging years. Our bodies slowly shift their proportions of "muscle mass" and "fat mass," losing some muscle or lean body mass and gaining some fat mass. Fat deposits tend, typically, to replace the cell tissue we lose in most parts of the body—the loss of as much as thirty percent of muscle mass during the middle years being offset by an increase in fat deposits. And too often, the new fat is deposited in the stomach and hip areas. Actually, a person typically reaches his maximum weight in his early forties and stays more or less the same until his late sixties, when he will be prone to weight loss.

The loss of up to thirty percent of our cells in muscle and soft tissue requires our metabolism to make adjustments. Older people have fewer cells burning energy, in short, and a decreased metabolic rate could mean a decreased blood flow. In drug therapy, physicians must remember this decrease in metabolism and blood flow in older people. Whether the decrease is simply an aging slowdown or is due to vascular disease, the circulation of drugs and nutrients is impeded. A loss of cellular mass also means a lowered water content in the body, so that a drug dosage resulting in a particular concentration in a young adult's system will result in a much higher concentration in an older person.

Drug therapy must also consider the muscle-fat shift during aging. Many drugs are fat soluble, which means that they linger in fat cells. In fat people, drugs cannot do their jobs as quickly as they do in lean people, and an elderly person who has a higher proportion of fat deposits than lean mass will retain a drug in his body longer than a younger person will. The effects of the drug will stay with him longer than with a lean person, and when a person is taking several drugs simultaneously, retention time and elimination time are very important for doctors to remember. In fact, drugs should be administered in quantities according to general health, body mass, height, and weight, rather than mere age.

Changes Affecting Drug Dosage

We find it increasingly difficult to maintain our youthful curves and contours as we age, and the reason is our body's general loss of lean mass. A certain amount of subcutaneous fat which is just underneath the skin is really part of the lean mass we lose, and without it, our bony features assume prominence. In addition to the loss of subcutaneous fat, the general dehydration of our tissues and years of muscle-flexing also contribute to our creases and wrinkles.

The loss of cell tissue in our organs, combined with our changes in size and blood flow, means that gradual adjustments must be made in the ways organs do their jobs. Our organs have tremendous reserve capacities, so even with a thirty percent tissue loss, they will not fail us—they just slow down a bit. The body is so well designed, it finds ways to compensate for the adjustments brought by age. Where drugs are concerned, the kidneys and the liver are preeminently important.

The kidneys are filled with microscopic structures called nephrons, highly specialized tubular systems that develop very early in life. Nephrons are structurally composed of glomeruli and tubules which are intimately interwoven with the capillaries of the circulatory system. The tubules of the nephrons eventually lead to the urinary ducts and the bladder and so in this close association between the nephrons and the capillaries, waste matter and excess salt is removed from the bloodstream and the proper pH (or acidity) of the blood is maintained along with an appropriate water level. The complex process requires differentiated cells that can sort out waste and filter it from the matter to be recycled and used by the body. Like all specialized cells, once these filtering cells of the kidney are developed, their numbers are set; we don't develop more of them. After maturity, we start to lose glomeruli and tubules and they are replaced with connective tissue, not by new filtering tissue. A young person's kidneys have approximately one million nephrons, but between the ages of 30 and 90 as much as a third may be lost. The result is that the amount of time the kidneys require to filter the waste from the blood or to return the blood to its proper salt balance and pH is significantly longer in elderly people than in young adults. Simply stated, the filtering rate of the kidney decreases with age. Since many drugs are filtered from the blood by the kidneys, it is this change in the filtering rate that means physicians must adjust dosages of drugs for the elderly.

Why does the kidney's filtering apparatus diminish with age? Perhaps the wear and tear theory of aging applies because dealing with waste matter day after day is inevitably and progressively harmful. Sometimes the waste becomes insoluble and is deposited in the kidneys, clogging up the nephrons and interfering with filtration from the blood to the urine. Kidney stones are a good example of insoluble waste and there are others such as immune complexes which, when deposits are found, may even lead to diseases such as glomerulonephritis and pyelonephritis. Arterial change is another factor affecting the aging kidneys, since a general thickening of the blood vessels occurs with aging. Although everyone's blood vessels stiffen and thicken at different rates during life, an increased rate of thickening is common in diabetes and for this reason, diabetics often develop kidney failure. High blood pressure is also associated with kidney malfunction, for then they are unable to rid the body of excess fluid.

Drinking plenty of water helps functional kidneys to stay clean and clear of insoluble waste: Water flushes the kidneys clean; clean kidneys flush the blood clean. A low back pain

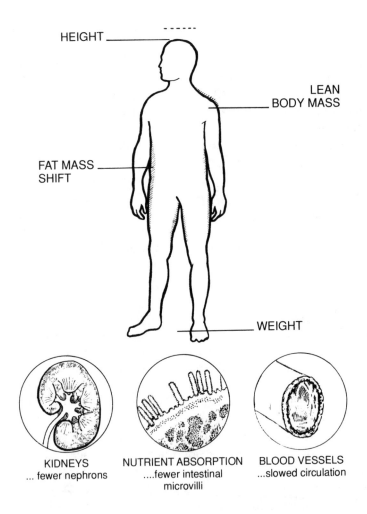

HEIGHT

LEAN
BODY MASS

FAT MASS
SHIFT

WEIGHT

KIDNEYS
... fewer nephrons

NUTRIENT ABSORPTION
....fewer intestinal
microvilli

BLOOD VESSELS
...slowed circulation

Figure 10 Aging changes affecting drug dosage: As we grow older our bodies respond generally more quickly to drugs, and retain them longer. Changes in height, weight, and muscle/fat proportions are part of the reason. Fewer nephrons in the kidneys and stiffer blood vessels slow the circulation of drugs; slightly smaller organs handle the drug less easily; absorption in the intestine, due to fewer microvilli, takes more time; and our tissues, slowly dehydrating, take up more of the available liquid. Changes in the nervous system can affect the autonomic respiratory response to some drugs.

often has nothing to do with the spine, but is, rather, the kidneys' call for help. They need water to unclog their nephrons.

Drug dosage is only one of the aging adjustments necessitated by age onset changes of the kidneys. All our bodily processes that rely on functional kidneys generally need a longer period of time to readjust in an elderly person. Homeostasis is a scientific word for the body's ability to adjust some of its systems to compensate for changes in others of its systems; the kidneys are prime regulators of homeostasis, or equilibrium. Blood pH, for example, is maintained within the narrow range of 7.35 to 7.45 and activities like vigorous exercise for long periods of time will make the blood more acidic. It is the kidney and pH sensors associated with the brain that work together to bring the pH back to its normal range.

In experiments using young and old volunteers who were given ammonium chloride, both groups registered increased blood acidity. It was found that the time needed for the return to normal acidity was almost twice as long in the old people as in the young. What that shows is that with the proper adjustments (such as allowing sufficient time) healthy kidneys can confront the challenges of filtration for us as we age. Homeostatic adjustments take a little longer in the elderly than in the young, but they certainly take place.

There is little change in the liver as we age. This organ, the largest gland we have, is so important that Mother Nature blessed it with the ability to regenerate, unlike the kidneys. Its size and function do not normally decrease until we are so elderly that we have become frail. Our liver is the organ that protects us from harmful substances in food and drink, working by rearranging the molecules of toxic substances so they become water soluble or mixed with bile, passing out of the body with urine and solid wastes. The liver screens most drugs for us and, for that matter, most of the things we ingest. As blood vessels emerge from the intestine carrying newly digested nutrients along with waste material, they form the portal vein that goes into the liver; the liver purges everything that is unwanted. It detoxifies the material before it goes to the rest of the body. That's why some drugs cannot be administered orally—the liver is so good at what it does, it will take the punch right out of a drug. Some drugs must be given intravenously or intramuscularly so they can reach the bloodstream without passing through the liver first. The liver manufactures bile, a substance which breaks down fats so that the lipase enzymes can then digest them, and it also transforms certain amino acids into proteins which serve as antibodies and other blood components. Still another of its tasks is to convert uric acid to the less acidic urea.

Cirrhosis, until recently, was thought of as the disease of alcoholics, but now it is known that people may develop cirrhosis of the liver without touching a drink. The problem is that their liver cells have lysed, or broken open, the cellular membranes ruptured. That can be caused by viral infection (hepatitis) as well as by too much alcohol. Efficient as it is, the liver can handle only so much alcohol; a flood of alcohol (and excessive amounts of iron supplementation or vitamin A) can cause liver cells to lyse. Although the liver can regenerate itself, there are limits—it won't do it forever and it will only go so far each time.

Many alcoholics (and heavy drinkers) have a distended abdomen that is the result of an inflamed, enlarged liver rather than a weight gain. "DT's" or shakes and tremors are a signal that the liver has given up and that toxins are being allowed into the bloodstream, homeostasis breaking down while the liver struggles to detoxify the alcohol. It is also a signal of imminent brain damage, and sometimes death.

Alcoholism is a self-limiting disease in the non-medical but literal sense because it usually leads to an early death. Alcohol is not a stimulant like caffeine, but rather, a depressant; when it is used to excess, it depresses life. The disease is not a major health problem of elderly people simply because most alcoholics do not live long enough to become elderly. By succumbing to their need for drink, alcoholics slowly commit suicide, assuming they do not die first in an automobile accident or from an angry argument leading to the use of a household firearm. Besides liver diseases, people who drink to excess tend to develop respiratory diseases, pharyngeal cancer, cardiovascular disease, organic brain syndrome, and, of course, nutritional deficiency. In the process of all this misery, they try, more often than not, and unintentionally, since they are enslaved to their disease, to destroy the lives of their families and friends.

Alcohol not only acts as a poor substitute food for alcoholics, it also inhibits the absorption of nutrients in the gastrointestinal tract. So alcoholics starve themselves, especially when their drinking takes the place of eating. Respiratory problems are caused by two effects of alcohol: It has a high rate of evaporation, so the resulting fumes cause injury to the delicate tissues in the lungs, and it depresses the central nervous system so the lungs and breathing fail to work at capacity. Alcohol sidetracks the neural instructions from the brain, interfering with their arrival in the lungs. Evaporation of alcohol is the reason a heavy drinker's breath gives him away. Additionally, the smell of aldehyde (a detoxification product from alcohol) seeps through an alcoholic's skin. Cardiovascular problems result from alcohol's continual depressing of the circulatory system, leading to clogged vessels and high blood pressure.

A recent study by Kenneth Borow of the University of Chicago found that three cocktail-sized drinks of scotch consumed at twenty-minute intervals reduced the left venticle's capacity of contracting and pumping blood out of the heart. The sobering part of the study: These results came not from middleaged or older persons; Borow's experimental subjects were healthy young men, all in their twenties.

Perhaps the most gruesome physical outcome of alcoholism is myelinolysis, the condition that results when the insulation around nerve cells dissolves. It is like multiple sclerosis which may be caused by viral infections and autoimmunity. The result of myelinolysis is cerebellar degeneration, also called organic brain syndrome.

Cigarette smoking, like excessive drinking, prevents the body from aging in good health. Among the many well-known harmful effects on the body from nicotine is the lung disease called emphysema. Black lung disease is the name coal miners gave to focal dust emphysema, a variation of the condition by which the alveolar sacs of the lungs are destroyed. The disease makes breathing difficult and can lead to kyphosis or barrel chest, since auxiliary thoracic muscles develop to aid in breathing. Emphysema is an aging disease, rarely striking people under 40, and its causes are pollutants like coal, dust, and cigarette smoke, and genetically, an inborn deficiency of antitrypsin which allows unrestrained enzyme destruction in the lungs. Smoking more than a pack of cigarettes daily for many years makes for severe cases of emphysema.

Gastrointestinal Aging Adjustments

Alcohol and nicotine are not the only drugs that have lingering effects in us as we age. The effects of most drugs may be prolonged by a diminishing rate of absorption in the gastrointestinal tract. Although healthy people do not normally lose the ability to absorb nutrients and drugs, the absorption may take a little longer when we are older—again, because of the body's generalized cell loss. The microvilli are cells of the intestinal walls, projections which provide additional surface areas for the exchange of nutrients. When we have fewer of them, we cannot absorb what we ingest as quickly as we once did, and that means that a small dosage of a drug can produce results that it takes larger doses to produce in young people. Moreover, when a drug affects the central nervous system, a small dose often has a qualitative difference in the elderly.

The central nervous system consists of cells, and it also

loses tissue mass as we age. The nerves' capacity for conducting sensory signals must therefore make adjustments, just as the other systems. At the same time, because muscle contraction ability also adjusts with age, older people's reflexes are slowed. A generalization we can make about elderly people is that their ability to cope rapidly with stress—mental or physical—is somewhat compromised. They simply cannot react as quickly as young people—but this is not to say the elderly cannot deal with stress. Although their blood flow, nerve conduction, and organ tissue mass may be only seventy-five percent of what it once was, they have an advantage over young people in one regard: They hold an increased percentage of experience, another aging adjustment in Mother Nature's wise planning. A lifetime of experience provides compensation for a diminishing physical capacity. The elderly may react to stress with more rationality than the young, if not as quickly.

The reason a combination of alcohol and tranquilizers can be lethal is that they are both sedatives, acting to depress the central nervous system. The central nervous system can be depressed to such an extent that not only will it stop instructing the lungs to breathe, but the diaphragm will also stop contracting so the person will die of asphyxiation.

Pressures accompanying aging and providing the need for adjustment, pressures such as the loss of a loved one, retirement, economic uncertainty, and loneliness, are met by many middleaged and older persons by a reliance on psychoactive drugs to help them cope. Because our society's system of advertising encourages self-medication, many older people seek not only their physician's advice but also his prescriptive sympathy, believing they cannot adjust without chemical assistance. At the same time, they consume non-prescription drugs, such as analgesics and laxatives, without the physician's awareness. Drugs, of course, work miracles, but one must not forget their harmful, pleiotropic potential. They may necessitate additional drugs for controlling unexpected effects: A person takes aspirin for his headache; the aspirin

causes gastric upset, so he takes an antacid; the antacid leads
to constipation so he takes a laxative. Another pleiotropic
effect of drugs is their high cost. It has been estimated that
elderly people buy one third of the drugs sold in the United
States, and, barring a major hospitalization, the cost of drugs
is the largest medical expenditure of elderly people. Taking
five or six or more different drugs at the same time is far from
being an uncommon practice, and often, the elderly pill-
poppers are completely unaware of the probable adverse
reactions they may experience. For one thing, the instructions
on the back of packaged non-prescription drugs are usually
directed, in size of print, to a younger person's eyesight.

"Misuse" and "abuse" have different meanings where
drugs are concerned. Normally, the word "misuse" describes
a failure to follow the instructions for prescription drugs.
"Abuse" is generally applied to illegal or illicit drugs and
alcohol. But whatever associations one makes with the two
words, there is no doubt about one thing: Misusing any drug
abuses good health.

When physicians prepare to prescribe medicine, they
usually ask a patient what other drugs he is taking. Since
drugs interact with each other to cause unwanted effects,
even aspirin or a glass of wine can affect the prescription the
physician prepares. And, because of the changes that occur
as we grow older—the decreases in blood flow, respiratory
adjustments, and organ efficiency—multiple drug consumption can have serious consequences.

Commonly Consumed Classes of Drugs

Following are some of the most often used medicines of our
society's drug culture. Common side effects are described,
along with some of the interactions that can be expected when
a drug is used at the same time with other drugs. It should be
remembered that all of them have heightened effects when
used by elderly people.

SEDATIVES and TRANQUILIZERS relieve anxiety and nervousness and are intended as temporary treatment—a period of a few days for a patient to take stock of his problems—not as a semi-permanent aid in facing reality. Far too many people believe they need the comforting effect of barbiturates after a trying time (such as a death in the family) rather than relying on their own emotional strength and the support of their close friends. It is a telling sign of our drug culture; the drug Nembutal is convenient in a world grown too fast-paced for religion and friendship. Unfortunately, many overworked physicians over-prescribe phenobarbital for patients who are all too eager to anesthetize themselves against a rough reality, and the result is addiction. Even less potent tranquilizers, such as Valium, can be habit-forming.

Sedatives such as Seconal, Dexamyl, and Nembutal decrease the effects of most other drugs taken simultaneously (with the notable exceptions of the antihistamines and alcohol, combinations which cause increased sedation). Tranquilizers such as Thorazine and Prolixin may dangerously impair heart function when taken along with quinidine or other antiarrhythmics. They steal some of L-dopa's potency, and they heighten the effects of antihistamines. Haldol may cause low blood pressure when it is taken at the same time as some antihypertensives, and with alcohol it may rob the brain of some of its function. With alcohol, Valium results in heavy sedation. Because sedatives and tranquilizers have even greater effects on elderly people who often take multiple drugs daily, accidents such as broken hips occur easily.

ANTIDEPRESSANTS are prescribed for serious depression (the most prevalent mental health disorder of elderly people) which usually shows physical manifestations such as appetite loss, weight loss, or lethargy. Unlike sedatives, antidepressants are used for extended therapy—weeks or months—and they produce side effects in most people, ranging from cardiac arrhythmias to low blood pressure. In men, they produce prostate problems. Although the depression may take several weeks to go away, the side effects are noticed immediately. Antidepressants such as Tofranil, Elavil, and Sinequan may also be prescribed for headaches, as well as for insomnia and some digestive disorders. If taken with alcohol, they can cause excessive intoxication.

MONAMINE OXIDASE (MAO) INHIBITORS are antidepressants which block nerve transmissions so that depression is not experienced. With caffeine, they cause high blood pressure; with antihypertensives, low blood pressure. Normal side effects from MAO inhibitors are dizziness upon changing position (such as getting up from bed), a dry mouth, constipation, difficulty in urinating, fatigue, and, sometimes, fainting, nightmares, and swollen legs. Longterm use of MAO inhibitors may lead to liver damage and they are quite dangerous for people with hypertension or heart disease. Even for healthy people, they may cause unpredictable blood pressure changes when taken with amphetamines, diuretics, and L-dopa.

HYPNOTICS, such as Placidyl and methaqualone (Quaalude), are habit-forming and are used to relieve anxiety and insomnia. They have profound effects on other drugs taken simultaneously: They decrease the effects of cortisone, aspirin, beta-blockers, and oral contraceptives; they increase the effects of antidepressants, antihistamines, MAO inhibitors, pain relievers, tranquilizers, sedatives, sleeping pills, and alcohol. Taken with anticoagulants, they may cause hemorrhaging.

ANTIHISTAMINES offset the flow of histamine (mucus—an initial immune response) in head colds, hay fever, and allergies, and they can help relieve motion sickness. Sold as such brands as Allerest, Chlor-Trimeton, Sudafed, Sinarest, Nytol, and Benadryl, the antihistamines produce the side effects of nausea, a dry mouth, nose, or throat, and drowsiness. If taken with alcohol, sedatives, tranquilizers, sleeping pills, or antidepressants, anti-histamines cause excessive sedation. What's more, they can intensify sunburn.

MUSCLE RELAXANTS (some of which are metaxalone, carisoprodol, and chlorphenesin) reduce spasms and cramps occuring after musculoskeletal and spinal injuries. They intensify the effects of anesthetics, central nervous system depressants, sedatives, tranquilizers, antidepresssants, antihistamines, and alcohol. Tobacco, on the other hand, inhibits their usefulness.

APPETITE SUPPRESSANTS, unfortunately, come with the pleiotropic effects of being habit-forming and causing nervousness, sleeplessness, and irritability. They are definitely not the best way to reduce calorie intake. Overdoses can cause comas, hallucinations, convulsions, or, less drastic, mood changes and a rapid heartbeat. They stimulate the brain's appetite control center, and with alcohol, caffeine, and MAO inhibitors, they increase blood pressure. With tranquilizers, sedatives, and antihistamines they can increase blood pressure dangerously.

COUGH SUPPRESSANTS affect the brain, inhibiting the nerve signals of the cough urge, so they can cause drowsiness, unsteadiness, and constipation in older people. In elderly men, difficulty in urinating and prostate enlargement are common side effects of cough suppressants containing chlophedianol, which is used as a local anesthetic and for dry coughs. Sedation results from simultaneous use with antihistamines, sleeping pills, tranquilizers, pain pills, muscle relaxants, and antidepressants. Dextromethorphan (contained in Dristan Cough Formula, Vick's Cough Syrup, and St. Joseph's Cough Syrup) is used for coughs in colds, bronchitis, and flus and may produce a drop in blood pressure, fever, and loss of consciousness when used with MAO inhibitors.

ORAL CONTRACEPTIVES regulate the menstrual period and the implantation of a fertilized egg and prevent the entry of sperm at the cervix. Women should never use these without a physician's guidance if they have fibrocystic breast disease, migraine headaches or seizures, asthma, hypertension, endometriosis, diabetes, or sickle cell disease. While taking them, they should not smoke cigarettes or use spinal anesthesia. Tobacco's effect on oral contraceptives may lead to strokes or heart attacks. Under normal circumstances, common side effects are brown skin blotches, itching, and fluid retention. Oral contraceptives sometimes cause blood clots in the legs, nausea and vomiting, bloating, headaches, and depression. Anticoagulants, anticonvulsants, antihistamines, and antiinflammatory agents, when taken at the same time as oral contraceptives, lessen the chance of their effectiveness.

ANTICHOLINERGICS help reduce digestive system spasms, but may cause confusion, a dry throat, rapid heartbeat, and constipation. Antidepressants, antihistamines, and haloperidol increase the effects of anticholinergics such as atropine (Donnagel, Contac), belladonna, and isopropamide (Combid).

Drugs for Parkinsonism (LEVODOPA (L-DOPA) and AMANTADINE) help restore the chemical balance for normal nerve impulse, reducing the tremors characteristic of Parkinson's disease. Levodopa also produces mood changes, diarrhea, and body odor. Haloperidol increases its effect; vitamin B_6 decreases it; MAO inhibitors team with levodopa to increase blood pressure. Amantadine is sometimes used to treat Type-A flu, as well as Parkinson's, and it causes appetite loss, purple skin blotches, fainting on changing position, and hallucinations. Alcohol increases the probability of fainting, and appetite suppressants cause nervous agitation with amantadine.

ANTACIDS come primarily from three drugs, aluminum hydroxide (Di-Gel, Mylanta, Rolaids, Maalox), calcium carbonate (Titralac, Tums, PeptoBismol), and sodium bicarbonate (Bromo Seltzer, Alka-Seltzer Antacid, Arm and Hammer Baking Soda). They act by neutralizing some of the stomach's hydrochloric acid and by reducing the digestive action of the enzyme pepsin. Used often for treating ulcers, they are also effective in helping the hyperacidity stemming from hiatal hernia, a condition that aging can worsen. Using them often produces the side effects of constipation, appetite loss, and belching; prolonged use can weaken the bones and result in too much calcium in the blood which can clog the kidneys or create kidney stones. Antacids lessen the effects of most other drugs being taken at the same time, particularly iron supplements, digitalis, anticoagulants, sulfa drugs, and vitamins A and C.

LAXATIVES, many of which are similar in action to antacids, are often excessively used by elderly people and are most beneficial for persons with heart conditions (since they can reduce straining from constipation, which is itself often caused by other drugs). Magnesium hydroxide, the ingredient in Milk of Magnesia, reduces the effects of anticoagulants, digitalis, iron supplements, and penicillin. Psyllium, the drug in Metamucil, has the same interactions, and, additionally, decreases the effects of most antibiotics and aspirin. Castor oil used simultaneously with antihypertensives and diuretics may cause low levels of potassium, while sodium phosphate (Sal Hepatica) and magnesium sulfate (Epsom Salts) may cause intestinal blockage when used with tetracycline. Mineral oil is an effective laxative, but its chronic use necessitates vitamin supplementation. Physical and psychological dependence often accompanies prolonged use of any laxative, and this is especially true of elderly people's use.

ANALGESICS, used to relieve pain, range from the mild acetaminophen (Tylenol, Vanquish, Sinarest, Excedrin, Datril) to the habit forming narcotic analgesics such as opium and morphine, to the steroids such as cortisone. Acetaminophen is used for slight pain and fever, and is thought to act on the hypothalamus, where the brain receives pain signals. It does not relieve inflammation or swelling, and may damage the liver and the kidneys. Long use can potentially cause anemia. With alcohol, acetaminophen causes drowsiness. With anticoagulants, there is danger of hemorrhaging—as is the case with aspirin, which is not only a pain reliever, but also an antiinflammatory drug used to relieve stiffness or the joint pain of arthritis. Aspirin contains sodium, and its side effects (besides the well known ones of stomach and intestinal irritation) may be nausea, heartburn, and ringing in the ears. Used with anticoagulants, cortisone, and alcohol, aspirin can facilitate bleeding and it potentiates ulcers. Antacids lessen aspirin's strength.

Ibuprofen, a fairly new antiinflammatory non-steroid drug sold as Motrin, Advil, Nuprin, Medipren, and Rufen, has become a popular choice for arthritis and menstrual pain. Although it often causes dizziness and headaches, for the most benefit it should be taken for several weeks. Taken simultaneously with aspirin, cortisone, or alcohol, ibuprofen can irritate the stomach and even cause ulcers. Taken for long periods of time, this drug (as well as Meclomen) has the potential for causing weight gain and even loss of vision and hearing.

Phenacetin, the analgesic in A.P.C. Tablets, Percodan, Fiorinal, and Sinubid, weakens the action of the body's prostaglandins, the early immune chemical messengers which are involved in fever and inflammation. Salicylate (contained in Mobidin and Arthropan) acts as a vasodilator, so it carries the danger of excessive bleeding, especially when used with other antiinflammatories, anticoagulants, cortisone, and alcohol.

Prednisone, triamcinolone, and cortisone suppress the

immune response and produce indigestion, thirst, and poor wound healing, as well as aggravating ulcers and bone loss. Their effect increases when used with aspirin, alcohol, and tobacco; it decreases when they are used with antihistamines and beta blockers; when used with digitalis and diuretics, cortisone reduces the body's potassium stores. The narcotic analgesics are those containing codeine, such as Darvon, Demerol, and Robitussin, or opium, methadone, and morphine. They block the signals of pain from reaching the spinal cord or the brain, and can cause dizziness, a flushed face, fatigue, urination difficulty, and, of course, addiction. They increase intoxication from alcohol and the effects of almost all other drugs.

ANTIHYPERTENSIVES such as clonidine (Catapres) and methyldopa (aldomet) are vasodilators, so they act to enlarge the arteries and to prevent fluid retention. They are used for treating high blood pressure and vascular headaches, and can produce lightheadedness when one changes postural position. Dizziness and drowsiness are also common results, as are enlarged breasts. Caffeine, a vasoconstrictor and antidepressant, weakens the effects of antihypertensives and alcohol intensifies them, causing low blood pressure. Some of them produce an irregular heartbeat when used with digitalis, and a dangerous heart rhythm with cortisone.

DIURETICS such as Aldactone also treat high blood pressure by helping the elimination of salt from the body fluid. However, headaches can result, along with vomiting and appetite loss. Like the antihypertensives, diuretics can lower blood pressure suddenly and excessively with alcohol and can cause irregular heart rhythm when taken with digitalis. With salt substitutes, diuretics may cause potassium levels to rise. *ANTIANGINAL* drugs such as cardizem and nifedipine (Procardia) reduce arterial pressure and facilitate the supply of oxygen to the heart. If they are used, though, with antihypertensives, beta blockers, diuretics, or alcohol, then hypotension can occur. The *ANTIARRHYTMICS* such as procainamide and quinidine correct heart rhythm disorders by delaying the nerve signals regulating heartbeat. Caffeine can make the heartbeat too rapid with antiarrhythmics, and tobacco can upset the regularity. Caffeine is the ingredient of vasoconstrictors such as Nodoz, Percodan, and Vivarin. Classified as a stimulant, caffeine has strong effects: it can cause nervousness, insomnia, and low blood sugar; it may cause or worsen fibrocystic breast disease; it decreases the effects of tranquilizers and alcohol; and it increases the effects of oral contraceptives, MAO inhibitors, and thyroid hormones.

BETA-ADRENERGIC blockers such as propanolol (Inderal), metoprolol (Lopressor), atenolol, and nadolol help to reduce angina and to control irregular heartbeats, lowering blood pressure and slowing blood vessel contractions and nerve impulses to the heart. They also reduce the strength of simultaneously used antihistamines and antiinflammatories, and heighten the effects of antihypertensives. When beta blockers and alcohol are used together, the blood pressure drops can be sudden and excessive.

ANTICOAGULANTS such as heparin are usually given in hospitals to reduce blood clots. A commonly prescribed oral anticoagulant is coumadin. A side effect often is gas and bloating. Most other drugs taken with an anticoagulant will increase its effect, a potential for serious bleeding. The new drugs for administration during a heart attack—streptokinase and TPA—belong in this category. Another new drug, lovastatin (sold as Mevacor) can reduce total cholesterol levels when it is used as an adjunct to a prescribed diet.

ANTIBIOTICS (penicillin, erythromycin, tetracycline, lincomycin, rifamycin, cephalosporin, neomycin, and the antifungal griseofulvin) prevent the growth and reproduction of bacteria and some fungi. Their main interactions are with each other, but it is not often that more than one or two are prescribed at the same time. Some of them are toxic to the liver—especially when alcohol is used with them, a combination that easily causes stomach irritation. Tetracycline increases the effects of lithium, digitalis, and anticoagulants, and it decreases the effects of antacids and oral contraceptives. Rifampin, used for tuberculosis and some other lung infections, decreases the effects of almost all drugs and with a few, such as alcohol and Isoniazid, it can damage the liver.

SULFA DRUGS, such as Bactrim are used to treat some bacterial infections, because they interfere with folic acid, a bacterial nutrient. Sulfa is hard on the kidneys, so much liquid should accompany them. Liquids containing vitamin C are not recommended, however, because vitamin C can heighten the kidney damage.

Chapter 6

Diet is for Life

The next time you're in a supermarket, pick up a ten pound bag of sugar. Hold it tightly against your body with one arm and continue your shopping. See how long you can hold the ten pound bag of sugar before you relent and drop it in your grocery cart.

A silly exercise? Of course. Why carry around a ten pound bag of sugar when you don't have to? It makes you tired. And that is exactly what being ten pounds overweight does—carrying extra weight around all the time, in all the daily movements of walking, climbing steps, getting up from a chair, or getting in and out of a car, makes you more tired than you should be. Many of the aches and pains people feel as they grow older would simply not exist if they were not overweight. Losing ten pounds brings overweight people a rejuvenation of energy which they probably did not know they had.

As we age into our middle and older years, we don't need to eat as much food as we once did. We require the most food during our growth periods, when we are children and teenagers, and as young adults we still require sufficient calories to maintain an energetic metabolic rate. But in middle age, our metabolism slows—we have fewer cells to maintain, our muscles and bones lose some of their mass, and our organs adjust their workload. A slower rate of metabolism means we require fewer and fewer calories. In fact, after the age of 30 our calorie needs decrease about five percent each decade. We can assist the body by adjusting the quantity of food we eat and scientific research illustrates that by improving the quality and variety of our diet we can retard many of the problems of aging.

We Americans are not noted for our moderation. We eat too much, and when we realize we are overweight we impulsively seek the details of an immoderate diet—maybe a "crash" diet or a fad diet consisting of fruit or a chalky powder and nothing else. Such a diet inevitably leads to illness, not because we don't get enough to eat, but because it leaves essential nutrients out. Our bodies must have variety—a balanced diet—in order to maintain the complex metabolic processes that keep us going. Some people enroll in two week "fat farms" (nowadays euphemistically called longevity or health enhancement centers), where they starve themselves by nibbling at tasteless food, buy jogging outfits, order a home exercycle, and consult daily with a nutritionist. Often, when they go home, they put the jogging suit away in a drawer and fix themselves a good meal.

"You Americans all saw your psychiatrists in the Sixties," says a British lady who visits the United States every few years, "but by the early Eighties, I noticed, you had stopped going to them. Now you have your nutritionists."

If we eat immoderately, it seems, we want also to lose our extra weight or bad habits in dramatic, immoderate fashion. A diet lasting for two weeks, however, or even three months or a year, has no value unless it is habit forming. A diet must be for life. The three important things to remember about a diet are: 1) it is for the rest of your life, 2) it must have variety, and 3) it must be regular.

The human body likes regularity; immoderation puts stress and strain on our homeostasis or equilibrium. The body feels comfortable sleeping at the same time in every twenty-four hour cycle; its good health prefers that exercise be regular; and its digestion functions more smoothly when meals are eaten at the same times every day. Going all day without eating and then gorging the body with a huge meal is asking the stomach to perform overtime—a form of physical stress.

Eating the same thing every day, no matter how nutritious it is, is to ask for trouble. Only through a balanced diet full of variety does the body obtain the vitamins and minerals it needs. The term malnourishment more properly describes the dietary habits of many Americans (both young and old) than the serious undernourishment of some Third World countries. Many young people in the United States are actually malnourished because their diets are top-heavy with fast food and soft drinks. Lacking the essential nutrients human beings require, they are nervous and high strung without knowing why. Many old people, too, are malnourished because they eat the same thing every day—tea and toast often is their staple due to many reasons such as loneliness, badly-fitting dentures, the need to watch pennies, or the effects of drugs they are taking. They become depressed and blame it on old age, not thinking that the reason might be their unbalanced diet.

Many middleaged people fall for faddish, trendy diet advice which abounds on bookstore shelves and magazine racks—usually remaining in vogue for about the length of time they claim is required for weight reduction. Sadly, people who are noticing changes of age in their bodies try such diets and often become ill before government agencies intervene and stop the quackery. A good diet contains variety, as spelled out in "Dietary Guidelines for Americans," a 1980 publication by the United States Department of Agriculture and Department of Health, Education, and Welfare, which warned against restricted diets and excessive vitamin supplementation. It recommended eating a variety of foods with adequate starch and fiber and avoiding large quantities of fat (particularly saturated fat) as well as cholesterol, sugar, sodium, and alcohol. The National Research Council of the National Academy of Sciences has recommended the increased consumption of fruits, vegetables, and whole-grain cereals, while stressing the dangers of large quantities of fatty foods in its report, "Diet, Nutrition, and Cancer." Also on the list of foods to avoid were salt- and smoke-cured foods and alcohol in immoderate consumption.

If we continue, in middle age, to eat the same quantities of food we ate in our teens and twenties, calories that are not needed for our reduced metabolism will be stored for future energy needs. The storage, of course, becomes fat if we fail to burn it off with exercise. We gain weight when this is the case, not an especially complex biological phenomenon: Too many calories mean a gain in weight and that is a fact at any age. Too few calories mean a weight loss or a loss in physical activity.

Adjustments in the Digestive System

As children, we have about two hundred and fifty taste buds on our tongues. We lose more than half of them as we age; very elderly people have only about ninety. A recent study of the olfactory ability of almost two thousand people of various ages from 5 to 99 reported that olfactory impairment need not be counted among the inevitable changes of age. Only half of the people in the study between ages 65 and 80 showed a decline in smell discrimination; those between 20 and 40 showed almost none; women were better smellers than men at all ages; and people who did not smoke had the best noses of all. A combination of causes most probably accounts for diminished powers of smell after age 65, including cell loss in the olfactory epithelium, some slight neuronal loss in the brain, and changing levels of neurotransmitters which carry impulses from one nerve ending to another.

Perhaps these changes in taste and smell explain why children disdain exotic foods and why, as adults, we seek— even crave—flavorful dishes. Perhaps Mother Nature is trying to tell us to look for quality in our food as we age instead of immoderate quantity.

Taste buds employ receptors for recognizing various molecules of nutrients—the same method of recognition used by drugs and hormones and the organs they stimulate. When sugar and salt molecules, for example, fit certain receptors on the taste buds, an electrochemical signal rushes to the brain. That is how we can tell if something is not sweet enough, or too salty.

Changes occur with age along the digestive tract, not only on the tongue. The movement of food from the esophagus into the stomach takes more time in people over 70 years old. The reason? Peristaltic contractions diminish as muscles in general adjust to a loss of tone and a reduction in stimulation by the nervous system. Another change occurs in the rate of regeneration of the esophageal epithelium. The passage of food brings wear and tear on the esophagus, and this is amplified by overeating. The process of repair and healing, by the formation of new cells, slows with age.

Hiatal hernia, previously mentioned in another context, is an esophageal condition that can become an age-related problem. If the esophagus is shorter than it should be, the stomach must reach up for its food and gastric juices find their way into the esophagus, causing heartburn. Less than ten percent of people under 30 years old feel the effects of this congenital problem, but up to 60 percent of people over 60 develop gastric leaks from hiatal hernias.

In the stomach, a slow thinning of the gastric glands and the stomach lining takes place as we age. This results in decreases in gastric secretions, further resulting in a decrease in absorption of some nutrients (particularly iron and vitamin B_{12}). A reduction in epithelial cell renewal, responsible for these changes in the aging stomach, also occurs in the intestine. It is, of course, in the small intestine where most of our nutrient absorption takes place.

Normally these changes along the digestive tract bring us a slight loss of digestive capacity; gastrointestinal disorders are not an automatic result of them, but the changes would seem to indicate a diet of highly nutritious food is best for the elderly; less food, but better food. This regimen meets well, too, the changing calorie requirements of older people.

Ever notice the advertising blitz, during the early evening television news shows, for laxatives and pain relievers? That's the time most old folks are watching and they make up the prime market for laxatives. Because of decreased muscle tone in the large intestine, and slowing motor function in the colon, food that is unused by the body moves somewhat more slowly in older people. They believe they are constipated, and therefore need a laxative. The slowing of elimination causes an increase in diverticular disease, sometimes associated with abdominal pain or inflammation, and possibly, cancer of the colon. These problems, including enteritis, occur in about nine percent of people under 50 but there is a greater than fifty percent chance when we're over 70. As we age there is even a change in our "microbial flora," the intestinal organisms that aid us in digestion and protect us from disease causing organisms. It appears that we lose some, like the lactobacilli which help us break down carbohydrates, and we gain some potentially pathogenic parasites, like fungi, as we grow older.

Just as a gain in weight is dangerous to our health, so is a rapid weight loss. Our bodies automatically adjust the activities of the organ systems to adapt to changes. Our bodies want to maintain the balanced physical well-being of homeostasis. If our blood pressure increases, for instance, the nervous system and the endocrine system make slight adjustments, resulting in the return of the blood pressure to its normal range and the brain tells certain hormones to try to balance the blood pressure change. In biology a physical change requiring a homeostatic adjustment is called stress. And normally, this stress is not detrimental; it keeps in proper tone our systems that cause readjustments. But unlike the normal stress that causes readjustments, the stress from too rapid a weight loss jolts the body—especially the aging

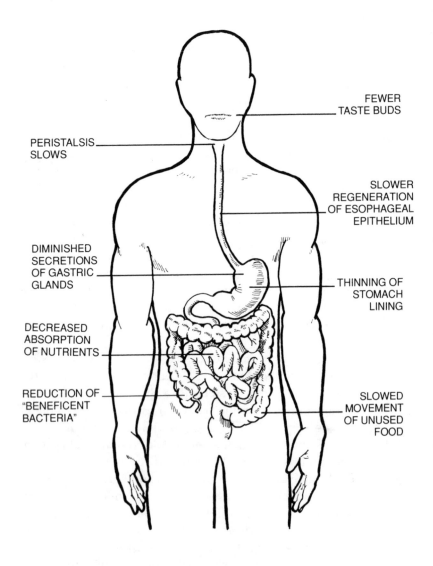

FEWER
TASTE BUDS

PERISTALSIS
SLOWS

SLOWER
REGENERATION
OF ESOPHAGEAL
EPITHELIUM

DIMINISHED
SECRETIONS
OF GASTRIC
GLANDS

THINNING OF
STOMACH
LINING

DECREASED
ABSORPTION
OF NUTRIENTS

REDUCTION OF
"BENEFICENT
BACTERIA"

SLOWED
MOVEMENT
OF UNUSED
FOOD

Figure 11 The changing digestive system

body. The aging body, already working hard to maintain homeostasis as our fat content is changing, also loses lean muscle mass, and the organs lose cell tissue. A sudden drop in nourishment compounds the changes requiring adjustments and can be stressful enough to send the body into physiological shock. Then it must use its reserves of sugar, glycogen, which it has stored in the muscles, and this speeds up the loss of muscle mass. Worse, the immune system, our great protector from disease, will lose function. In short, by dramatically reducing our nourishment, we compromise the body just as surely as when we go without sleep, expose ourselves to infection, or suffer a major injury.

The Essential Nutrients

Nutrients, according to the dictionary, are substances that keep a person, plant, or animal alive and well. Seven types of food keep us alive and (it is hoped) well: proteins, carbohydrates, fats, vitamins, minerals, water, and roughage. While water and roughage are not usually thought of as nutrients, they meet the definition because they are essential in keeping us alive and well.

PROTEIN gives us the amino acids our cells use to build, through DNA's instructions, our own proteins. Bodily proteins are very personal things and we always make our own, needing about twenty amino acids to make the proteins we must maintain for the body's well being. Although we manufacture half of these (the nonessential amino acids) from other foodstuffs, we must eat protein for the essential amino acids, for we do not synthesize them on our own. A protein deficiency at any age means we cannot make new cells for structural growth and repair; we cannot make the hormones we need for proper organ function and communication; we cannot make neurotransmitters to carry brain signals; and we cannot make antibodies to fight disease.

Vegetarians need to eat an inordinately large quantity of plant protein to obtain their essential amino acids. Although found in vegetables, grains, and wheat, the concentrations of the essential amino acids are much higher in animal meat. Dairy products, eggs, meat, and fish not only serve as rich protein sources, but also as good suppliers of many essential vitamins and minerals. Research has shown neither a difference in protein digestion nor in protein requirements between young and old people. What is different with age is the rate of absorption of some amino acids—a young body absorbs more, faster.

CARBOHYDRATES, the sugars and starches, provide our source of energy for all the chemical reactions within our cells. Without an adequate carbohydrate supply, the body uses the structural proteins for its energy needs. Our cellular power plants (the mitochondria) "burn" glucose and make ATP (adenosine triphosphate) which carries energy to each and every site where chemical reactions occur and which is fundamentally necessary for the synthesis of DNA. Sugar, molecularly known as a saccharide, comes in several molecular forms. Glucose is a monosaccharide and sucrose (table sugar) is a disaccharide—a molecule of glucose hooked to a molecule of fructose. Fructose, a sugar in fruits, is another simple sugar—a monosaccharide. Starch, the sugar in potatoes, pasta, corn, and rice, is a polysaccharide, many sugar molecules hooked together forming a chain of sugars. Humans and the other animals do not make sugar in our bodies; carbohydrates are made only by plants and so we completely depend on plants for our energy needs—they keep us alive and they keep alive the animals we use as protein sources.

Besides meeting our immediate and continuing cellular energy needs, sugar is stored in our muscles and in our liver in the form of glycogen, another starch. It is released when we need it for physical strain or when the amount of glucose in the blood drops. It is the glycogen stores in the meat of wild animals that tastes "gamey" to us. Wild animals get more exercise than domestic animals, thus, they have more glycogen in their muscles.

The difference between young and old people in the digestion and absorption of carbohydrates is so marginal that we can say there is none.

Fruits and vegetables, of course, give us vitamins and minerals along with carbohydrates. And they give us *ROUGHAGE* or cellulose—a polysaccharide that we cannot digest. But roughage (or fiber, as it is often called today) assists in the digestion of other nutrients by providing the bulk which aids the movement of food through the intestine. Roughage helps our nutrients in their journey to "absorption sites" in the intestine so we can make the most of them.

Refined foods are devoid of roughage. Marie Antoinette began a trend when she said, "Let them eat cake," a trend which altered the normal diet away from rough foods to refined foods. People wanted to eat light, fluffy cakes like Marie Antoinette ate, but you cannot make a white cake with whole wheat flour. People demanded refined, white flour to such an extent that all roughage was removed from the diet, and most modern stomach aches began. The fact is that our intestines need roughage. Indeed, throughout history the mammalian intestine evolved with a steady diet of roughage, grew accustomed to it, and it is only recently, in historical perspective, that we have asked our bodies to cope without it. Fortunately for us today, fiber is in vogue for everyone, including the elderly. And it is especially good for the elderly because it may help to stimulate the depressed peristaltic activity in the gastrointestinal tract. How much roughage we need is an individual matter. Like vitamin A, too much roughage presents problems and too little is no good either. The amount that facilitates intestinal function is different for all of us—too little can cause constipation and too much can lead to diarrhea. Diverticulosis can result from either too much or too little.

Some *FATS* or lipids (not a lot) are essential for us. Plants have the ability to make carbohydrates and fats, and while we are dependent on plants for our carbohydrate requirements, we can make some but not all of our fats. Fat is a concentrated form of energy and efficient, at that, for storing energy. It carries twice the number of calories per ounce as carbohydrate. The type of fat most commonly stored in the fat cells is triglycerides. When we need our reserve of triglycerides for energy, it is enzymatically converted into chemical forms that enter the energy cycle.

An interesting study by Ulf Smith of Sweden provides scientific evidence that a paunch is as unhealthful as it is unsightly. Fat cells in the area of the abdomen metabolize more rapidly than fat cells in other parts of the body, and, therefore, they release more fatty acids into the blood. The more fat cells in the abdomen, the higher the fatty acid concentration in the blood, and that leads to elevated triglyceride levels in the liver and impaired utilization of the body's glucose.

There are some essential fatty acids (just as there are essential amino acids) that we cannot make by ourselves. Vegetable oil (polyunsaturated fats) supplies us with the essential fatty acid we need for cell structure and maintenance, among other functions. We also need fatty acids for our production of prostaglandins, hormones which help to maintain our blood platelets and the contraction ability of the smooth muscle cells of our blood vessels and heart. Fatty acids appear to have something to do with the proper functioning of the nervous system and the perception of pain. So, while we need them for good blood circulation, good heart function, and proper nervous system function, there is a delicate balance involved. The combination of too much animal fat and too little fatty acid from vegetables may lead to cardiovascular disease. The American Heart Association recommends in its "prudent diet" that we reduce fatty foods to about thirty percent of our total calories, use skimmed milk instead of whole or even lowfat milk, cut down on fatty meats and eggs, and eat more fruits, vegetables, grains, poultry, and fish.

Many studies suggest that vegetables provide a safer source of dietary fat than does beef. The body needs cholesterol, a precursor of many hormones, and it needs unsaturated fats as the raw materials for making cholesterol, but excessive levels of cholesterol can clog the blood vessels by the formation of atherosclerotic plaques, the cause of coronary heart disease. The Harvard School of Public Health published in 1985 the results of its diet-heart study of Irish Bostonians, showing that a high intake of polyunsaturated fatty acids (the sort that comes from vegetables) and a low intake of saturated fatty acids and cholesterol (the sort obtained from beef, eggs, and whole milk) reduced mortality from coronary disease. Another study, this one from the Netherlands, illustrates how vegetables help us age by retarding heart disease. The researchers amassed evidence that a diet high in vegetables reduces the body's ratio of serum total cholesterol (the so called "low density lipoproteinbound" variety of cholesterol implicated in atherosclerosis) to the safer high density lipoprotein cholesterol.

Cholesterol-induced plaques in the blood vessels insidiously form during childhood and our adult years. The best time to reduce intake of saturated fats and cholesterol is not when we are old, but when we are still young. Any day, however, is a good time to begin. We should be wary of animal fats and moderate our consumption of vegetable oils.

There are very few differences between young and old people in the digestion, absorption, or requirements for fat.

A well balanced diet provides the thirteen essential *VITAMINS*: vitamins B_1, B_2, B_6, B_{12}, vitamin C, niacin, folacin, pantothenic acid, and biotin which are water soluble; and vitamins A, D, E, and K which are fat soluble. In recent years, many nutritionists, physicians, and health food advocates have recommended taking megadoses of various vitamins. They have heard about research showing that certain vitamin deficiencies in rats lead to graying of hair, reduced sexual activity, and a decreased life span. Apparently, these people have not considered that (1) the experiments were done with rats, not with people, and (2) dietary deficiencies caused the vitamin deficiencies. A balanced diet contains the thirteen essential vitamins; there is no need for excessive vitamin supplementation. Megadoses of anything can be unhealthful for the body and wasteful for the wallet.

What does a vitamin do? It normally acts as a middleman in an enzymatic chemical reaction. Thus, vitamins are often referred to as coenzymes. The B-complex vitamins, for instance, position a particular electron of a molecule so that it is in place for a reaction to occur successfully. When an enzyme's function is to join a molecule of glucose to a phosphate molecule, a vitamin moves the electron of the phosphate molecule to the vicinity of the glucose. Thus, vitamins are instrumental in the chemical binding of molecules, the fundamental activity in our bodies.

Some of them, like vitamin A, have a hormone-like activity. They stimulate cell growth by binding to specific receptors within the cell. Vitamin D and its stimulation of bone formation is another example of hormone-like activity. Some vitamins have a garbage collection function, acting as traps for free radicals of oxygen. Vitamins C and E head this list. Others play important roles in wound healing, resistance to infection, blood clotting, and vision.

VITAMIN A is in green vegetables, carrots, tomatoes, milk, butter, fortified margarine, and cheese. An excess can lead to headaches, skin peeling, bone swelling, loss of appetite, and hepatitis. A deficiency can lead to visual defects, blindness, and even cancer, according to a recent study in Great Britain. Although inconclusive, the study makes a good point: A vitamin, just as a drug, is nothing to play with; a vitamin imbalance can interfere with hormonal functions. Vitamin therapy is for a physician to prescribe as a result of a clear nutritional deficiency.

The *VITAMIN-B COMPLEX* is in pork and other meats, vegetables, eggs, dairy products, and whole grain cereals. Deficiencies lead to blood and nervous disorders (including anemia and muscular convulsions), dermatitis around the eyes, and kidney stones. This is especially true of a vitamin B_{12} deficiency. Megadoses of vitamin B_6 (pyridoxine) have been associated with nerve damage; deficiencies of vitamin B_1 (thiamine) may cause increased anxiety or depression. Vitamin B_2 (riboflavin) aids in oxidation of the tissues and its deficiency may result in lesions of the mucus membranes.

VITAMIN C is in fresh citrus fruits, salad greens, green peppers, and tomatoes. A deficiency causes scurvy, the traditional disease of sailors before they realized they should pack some oranges on board ship. Not abundant in processed foods, vitamin C helps in the biochemical synthesis of amino acids for the formation of collagen, cartilage, bones, and teeth. It seems to help the immune system in protecting us from viruses, but no one has established why; and it is an anti-oxidant, protecting cells from free radicals.

Even vitamin C has its dangers, however—an excess can lead to kidney problems. People who have been taking megadoses of vitamin C should not stop abruptly because the body could develop scurvy, sensing a "deficiency" of its customary level of the vitamin.

VITAMIN D, which helps us absorb calcium, is in eggs, dairy products, and cod-liver oil. A deficiency can lead to rickets and other bone disorders and thus is being studied these days as a potential weapon against osteoporosis. An excess leads to diarrhea, weight loss, and kidney damage.

VITAMIN E is in green vegetables, shortenings, margarine, and seeds. Like vitamin C, it prevents cell damage by capturing free radicals. A deficiency may lead to anemia or cancer; an excess does not appear to be toxic. Although animal experiments have given vitamin E a reputation for increasing physical and sexual activity, its potential for human beings is not by any means understood.

VITAMIN K is in green leafy vegetables, cereals, fruits, and meats. Since it aids in blood clotting, a deficiency can lead to severe bleeding and internal hemorrhaging. An excess does not appear to be harmful.

NIACIN is found in liver, lean meats, grains, and beans. A deficiency can lead to skin and gastrointestinal ulcers and nervous disorders. An excess causes itching and a burning feeling around the neck, hands, and face.

PANTOTHENIC ACID is in most foods. Only serious malnutrition results in its deficiency, which causes fatigue and impairs coordination.

FOLACIN is in beans, green vegetables, and whole wheat products. A deficiency leads to anemia, diarrhea, and other gastrointestinal problems.

BIOTIN is in beans, vegetables, and meats. Its deficiency leads to fatigue, depression, dermatitis, and muscular pain. No harm is known to result from an excess.

There are no dramatic differences between young and old in vitamin requirements. A balanced diet provides an adequate supply of vitamins, so vitamin supplementation should not be necessary in the absence of disease, malnutrition, or chronic use of drugs. Of concern to the frail elderly is absorption of vitamins through the stomach and intestine, a nutritional problem accompanying the gastrointestinal disease, gastritis.

MINERALS make up between five and seven pounds of an adult person's weight. Six "macroinorganic" minerals—sodium, potassium, calcium, magnesium, chlorine, and phosphorus—make up most of this poundage. The "microinorganics," iron, zinc, iodine, copper, fluorine, selenium, and several others, are essential also. We must get them from our diets.

Minerals generally have two main roles. Like vitamins, they serve as intermediaries in chemical reactions. They help maintain bone structure, teeth, and muscle contraction ability.

CALCIUM, PHOPHOROUS, AND FLUORINE are important for our bones and teeth. Their deficiency can stunt growth and lead to demineralization of bones, muscular convulsions (charley horse), osteoporosis, and can increase tooth decay frequency. We get calcium and phosphorus from milk, cheese, dark green vegetables, meat, and poultry. We get fluorine from seafood and fluorinated drinking water.

POTASSIUM which comes from milk, meats, and fruits, is important for muscular and nerve function.

IODINE is an important element of thyroid hormones. We get it from vegetables and dairy products as well as from seafoods.

IRON comes from eggs, lean meats, beans, whole grains, and green leafy vegetables. It is necessary in our formation of hemoglobin, the constituent of blood that carries oxygen throughout the body. Low levels of iron mean "tired blood," resulting in muscular weakness, anemia, and low resistance to infection. Too much iron can cause cirrhosis of the liver.

MAGNESIUM prods enzymes into protein synthesis; it comes from green leafy vegetables and whole grains.

SELENIUM, in seafood, meat, and some grains, seems to assist vitamin E's antioxidant activity.

ZINC is a constituent of digestive enzymes and other enzymes that direct nucleic acid metabolism. It comes from nearly all of our food. A deficiency can mean stunted growth, small sex glands, and immune deficiency. We need *SODIUM* and *CHLORINE*, which we get from table salt, to form and control our gastric juices and for nerve function. If we do not get salt, we can experience muscle cramps and even apathy; too much, of course, increases our blood pressure.

WATER is an essential part of our diet. Besides the obvious source, it comes from most solid foods and liquids. Its roles are to dissolve and transport nutrients within the body, to regulate our temperature, and to aid in many metabolic reactions. It serves as a purgative, too, flushing out toxins and waste matter. Without it we would dehydrate and die. Too much of it, ironically, causes headaches and high blood pressure.

Vitamin and Mineral Supplements or a Balanced Diet?

Many people who lose weight rapidly by dramatically reducing the amount of food they eat try to compensate with vitamin supplementation. They should remember that vitamins alone do not supply the essential nutrients; we must have protein, carbohydrates, fats, roughage, and water, along with vitamins and minerals. Recent research in nutrition has not disproved our mothers' advice: A balanced diet is the best assurance of getting an adequate supply of vitamins and all the essential minerals.

Widespread vitamin deficiencies simply do not exist in the United States today. Even with so many of us relying on fast food much of the time, vitamin deficiencies are not so strikingly evident as they were at the turn of our century. What does exist today is called "sub-clinical" vitamin deficiency, and we have sophisticated ways to detect it.

A test of lymphocytes (white blood cells) indicates malnourishment. In a normal measure 1500 lymphocytes are present. If a person's count drops under 1000 he is not properly nourished. Another test zeroes in on vitamin A. The presence of vitamin A stimulates the liver to produce a binding protein to pick up the vitamin—a low level of this protein in the blood indicates the vitamin deficiency. Still another test uses disease antigens. We make antibodies against common childhood diseases like chicken pox and measles. When disease antigens are inserted under the skin the antibodies should rush to the attack. If there is a delayed reaction, however, a person is probably malnourished.

Nutritional deprivation, or caloric restriction, is a research topic making headlines these days. The idea is that by eating less, we will live longer. There is some truth in the premise, but there are also some inherent problems with restricted diets. One should not stop eating after reading only the headlines. Indeed, an abrupt decrease in nourishment in middle age could very well shorten one's life, according to some scientists.

For one thing, the bulk of nutrition research is by animal experimentation—rats and mice. While rats are almost as biologically complex as human beings are, their living conditions and social arrangements are so different from ours that research findings can only be suggestive, certainly not definitive. Nutritional experimentation with human subjects is not possible in Western society. Severe restrictions in the diet of an elderly nursing home patient, even voluntary, is unthinkable. Social politics often makes it difficult for scientists even to study ethnic genetic differences among people.

Clive McKay, a scientist working at Cornell University

almost fifty years ago, found that when diet was restricted early in a rat's life and for a relatively short period, say, a week or so, the rat's life was prolonged by as much as a year, although its growth was somewhat retarded. For a rat which normally lives two to three years, that represented a twenty-five to thirty percent leap in longevity. More recent research, including that of Morris H. Ross of the Institute for Cancer Research in Philadelphia, has added to McKay's work. It appears that moderate reductions in feeding at any stage of a rat's life can add months to its life. Dr. Ross confirmed that nutritional deprivation during a rat's early days can lengthen its life, and he goes so far as to say that our adage, "We are what we eat," should be revised to "We are what we ate." But he has found that food reductions in middle and old age can shorten life span unless they are very moderate reductions. Some of his studies indicate that restricted diets of high protein probably prolong life but increase the chances of tumors and stunted development.

Roy Walford, a gerontologist at UCLA, extended these studies to mice, another mammal with a biological makeup paralleling that of human beings. He showed that mice on restricted diets gained an improved immune system defense. Their immune systems responded more rapidly when challenged with antigens, produced fewer self-destructive autoantibodies, and, in mice susceptible to tumor formation, inhibited such tumors. Caloric restriction has also been reported to result in diminished collagen cross-linking and decreased post absorptive cholesterol levels.

It is clear from these studies that eating less was better for the health of rodents, but a group of researchers at Harvard University disagree with the interpretation that the restricted diets increased the maximum life span of the mice. These scientists point out that laboratory mice and rats have traditionally been fed a heavy diet selected specifically for rapid reproduction and growth. You can do more laboratory experiments for your money when your mice are propagating quickly, yielding multiple offspring. According to the Harvard interpretation, the rich diet the laboratory animals usually received was actually shortening their life span, although no one realized it. The more recent investigations with caloric restriction, the Harvard scientists say, merely rediscovered the maximum life span of the mice under non-laboratory conditions. The restricted diet, it turns out, was really a normal diet. When the laboratory mixture for rapid growth was reduced to moderate proportions it became more like a normal diet and it prevented the premature onset of disease.

What is the relevance of all this for human beings? A fair interpretation is that a diet that keeps us lean and physically active will help us live to our genetically determined maximum life span. In fact, some human studies show lower mortality for people who are lean in their twenties and then gain about ten percent in weight during middle age. There are equivocal figures in other reports, though, showing longer lives for people whose weight is always slightly below average.

In Spain, E. A. Vallejo conducted a study a few years ago using nursing home patients over the age of 65. Half the people ate a normal institutional diet every other day, but restricted themselves to milk and fresh fruit on alternate days. After three years, the other half of the people, who ate the normal diet every day, had a death frequency twice that of the milk and fruit group. Vallejo's report also showed that the normal diet group spent twice as much time in the infirmary as the alternate day dieters.

Are vegetables and fruits the perfect foods? Answering such a question is not as simple as might be expected. Our food comes from Mother Nature with its own dangers and with its own protection against dangers, too, according to some studies by Bruce Ames of the University of California at Berkeley. Plants have natural defenses against disease and insects, and some of these defenses, it appears, are harmful to us. Dr. Ames has shown that plants have natural fungicides to prevent their fruit from producing mold, and they have natural insecticides for protection against bugs. These substances, "natural carcinogens," protect the plants but can be dangerous to us when we eat them. Likewise, many cooking processes produce carcinogenic compounds. A charcoal broiled steak, for example, has many types of carcinogens on it: unburned hydrocarbons from the charcoal, oxidized fat (that provides so much flavor), and even the meat's sugars, proteins, and amino acids, as they caramelize from the heat. We need to know more about these natural troublemakers, more about their real risk to us, so we can remove them from our dietary habits or, at least, remove the risk.

Dr. Ames's findings certainly do not mean we should stop eating fruits and vegetables. Our own defenses against natural carcinogens have evolved with the rest of our human composition. And the same plants which carry dangers carry other substances, vitamins, and minerals, which we use for defense. Our own defenses against carcinogens include the shedding of skin and the turnover of cells of our stomach lining and other parts of the digestive system. Incoming carcinogens react with these cast-off cells before they can penetrate to lower cellular levels. The way many carcinogens harm us is by producing free radicals of oxygen which can damage DNA's integrity, not to mention other cellular components. Still another defense is our enzymes, such as superoxide dismutase, which trap free radicals of oxygen before they create much mutation. Plants kindly provide us natural protection by supplying dietary antioxidants such as vitamin E, beta-carotene, selenium, glutathione, and vitamin C. These substances and other enzymes (such as catalase and peroxidase) trap and destroy free radicals. Animal studies using dietary antioxidants have shown life extensions, but the investigators admitted that the animals lost weight during the experiments, so the longer life might be due to caloric restriction.

Another example of the dangers inherent in massive doses of vitamins applies to the dietary antioxidants. In a study of people over the age of 65 who took megadoses of vitamin E daily, increased mortality was shown. Did they die

early because of vitamin toxicity or because they were unhealthy to begin with, a situation leading to their intake of
vitamin E? Scientists cannot be sure either way, but one point
is clear: There is simply not enough evidence to support
vitamin supplementation as a way to extend life.

There is strong evidence, however, that eating more fish
can retard heart disease, and therefore extend life, since
heart disease kills more people than any other cause. Researchers in the Netherlands followed eight hundred and
fifty-two middleaged men who in 1960 were healthy and free
of signs of coronary heart disease. By 1980 seventy-eight of
the men had died from coronary heart disease and among
those who ate fish once or twice a week the mortality rate was
fifty percent lower than among the men who never ate fish.
The researchers also point to Eskimos and natives of Japan,
habitual fish eaters, who have higher levels of high density
lipoprotein cholesterol in their blood and lower levels of total
cholesterol and triglycerides than is the case in red meat-rich
Western societies such as ours.

It seems far more advisable to increase one's intake of
fish, vegetables, fruits and cereals—for the purpose of retarding disease and retaining good health—than to waste money
on products such as Gerovital-H3, a mild antidepressant
containing procaine and hydrochloric acid and claimed to
extend life by no one except its own promoters. The United
States Food and Drug Administration ordered another of the
life extension gimmicks off the health food store shelves in
April, 1985. Known as DHEA, dehydroepiandrosterone is a
steroid hormone plentiful in our bodies when we are young
but declining as we age. No human experiments with DHEA
are of record, but in mice, the administration of DHEA
decreases the incidence of breast cancer, delays immune
dysfunction, and inhibits tumors. Again, these effects may
result from caloric restriction since the hormone makes the
mice lose weight. Until there is scientific data on human use
of DHEA, no one advises its consumption except those who
want to sell it.

Nutritional Needs and the Individual

Nutrient requirements depend on many factors besides age. As individuals, we differ genetically—each person possessing a unique mix of enzymes that go to work on food to extract nutrients. A muscular, physically active lumberjack may get slightly less protein from a steak or a halibut than his wife, a petite piano player, simply because her enzymes may be more numerous than his or they may work more efficiently. Age, sex, size, and physical activity all play important roles in our nutrient needs.

The way a particular nutrient is "packaged" by Mother Nature can affect its availability to us. Iron in meat and iron in cereal differ in their availability to us since our digestive systems have more in common chemically with animals than with plants. Our enzymes are more in tune with animal meat than with the complex carbohydrate chemistry of plants, and so we extract iron from meat more easily than we do from grains—although we can certainly get what we need if we persevere along without meat. Iron is so important to us that our bodies recycle it to an extent. When red blood cells die we do not lose all of the iron they contain—we extract it from the dying cells and use it again.

Disease and physical or mental trauma affect proper nutrition at any age and so do loneliness and apathy. Emotional upset can cause people to stop eating or to eat irregularly or inadequately. The condition of many a cancer patient worsens if he does not eat because without proper nutrition, the body is that much weaker against disease. It hardly needs saying that physical immobility and unsanitary conditions can lead to malnourishment. Poverty affects nutrition and being alone can lead to seriously harmful eating habits—especially among the elderly. Poverty usually means cold and damp substandard housing, and a lack of food refrigeration.

Drugs, as discussed in the last chapter, affect nutrition. An example is the antibiotic, tetracycline, that interferes with our absorption of calcium from dairy products. Excessive consumption of depressants like alcohol and sedatives interfere directly with digestion by slowing peristalsis in the intestine. Mineral oil can rob the body of vitamins A, E, D, and K, and oral contraceptives containing estrogen have been reported to cause clinical folate deficiencies. Aspirin decreases the body's absorption of vitamin C. Vitamin B_6 (pyridoxine) in a normal diet helps the immune system produce antibodies and it assists in protein metabolism, but in some persons taking massive doses, it has impaired nerve conduction and muscle coordination and it has actually killed neuronal cells.

As we age, a gradual decrease in the volume and the concentration of our gastric secretions—the digestive enzymes—means we have a harder time, or require a greater amount of time, obtaining our essential nutrients. Many sedentary elderly people become preoccupied with constipation, sometimes becoming physically and psychologically dependent on laxatives. The decrease in intestinal peristalsis, along with a lack of exercise, is responsible. The lack of exercise must be emphasized. We can retard the decline of digestive activity by exercising regularly.

Chapter 7

Appearance: Skin, Hair, and Teeth

As we age, we spend more time and money trying to retard not the changes taking place in our digestion, but the obvious changes in our skin and in our hair. We see these changes, after all, on a daily basis but we become aware of digestive system changes only sporadically, such as the midnight bout of heartburn. Culturally, we tend to equate youth and good health with appearance rather than with internal homeostasis. This does not totally miss the mark; appearance certainly can be an outward display of the state of health that is within. It is equally true, however, that wrinkling skin and thinning hair have nothing to do with health—they are physical, inevitable changes of age. The 90-year old lady in the mountains of Ecuador probably gives the outward appearance of a dried prune but she continues to make her way up and down and around those rocky village paths, out in the sharp wind and the bright sunlight of the high Andes. Whatever her appearance, she's still actively living her life. She's not supine in a dark hospital room, the only sound the gurgling, bubbling respirator tubed into the wall at the head of her bed. And she's 90.

Our appearance is so important to us that we expend great amounts of our precious time fretting about looking old. Mind you, not growing old, but looking old. Aging skin and aging hair affect us psychologically far more than they affect us biologically, yet we spend vast amounts of money, in

Western society, trying to look younger than we really are. Plastic surgery these days is a blanket term covering more than facial reconstruction for cosmetic reasons. Now we may reshape the body's contours, and a new procedure called suction lipoplasty removes fat cells from under the skin by the use of a hose connected to a sort of vacuum cleaner. It is proving effective for the removal of women's "jodhpurs" and men's "love handles," and for breast sculpture. Responsible plastic surgeons advise their customers though, that the procedure creates dangerous shifts of metabolism such as "contour ripples" and the unpredictable flow of fluid into the newly sculpted areas. Our society's priorities being what they are, these dangers of cosmetic surgery most likely will soon become the object of more research dollars than our hapless disease eradication struggles.

Plastic surgery depends for its success on the capacity of the skin to expand. When a hollow silicone "baggy" is inserted under the skin and then filled with saline to produce a desirable contour, it stretches the surrounding tissue. As we age, the skin loses some of its capacity to expand and too-rapid stretching may leave dermal scars (stretch marks) or the skin may actually split. Perhaps one of the best uses of plastic surgery has been the development of hair transplants, the replacement of bald patches of the scalp with hair-bearing grafts.

Certain drugs used for treating high blood pressure have caused hair growth, strangely enough, in about twenty percent of the people using them. They are now being marketed as a cure for baldness. We will see.

Science, alas, has little knowledge of the basic biological mechanisms underlying our aging skin and our aging hair, but all evidence points to inevitable changes, regardless of what lotions we rub on ourselves. Makeup can cover it up, but the changes are still there, for the primary reason behind wrinkling skin and thinning hair appears to be genetic. A secondary reason is, simply, years of accumulated exposure to the elements.

Cobblestones, Honeycombs, and Collagen

Our skin, the largest and heaviest of our organs, weighs about six pounds—that is, the skin of an average sized adult person. It contains about three thousand square inches of surface area and receives about a third of the body's circulating blood. In thickness it can vary from about one-fiftieth of an inch in an eyelid to about one-third of an inch in soles and palms. The human epidermis is a multi-layered system of cells, each one constantly on the move from the innermost layer to the skin surface where we shed them. Mother Nature has been kind to us, giving us this permanent, unnoticeable sloughing off of our skin. Some other species, such as snakes and birds, lose their entire skin covering or molt their feathers in one periodic heave, not always an easy chore. We have a better arrangement: Our skin cells originate deep within our covering, fill themselves up with a protein (keratin) and begin their journey up to the surface, forming layer upon layer of skin cells. At the surface, they are already dead cells and they fall off or exfoliate.

The time it takes for new skin cells to journey up through the skin all the way to their exfoliation has been the subject of investigation to see if there is a difference in young and old skin cell renewal. A way to measure the transit time of skin cells is to stain the layers and then to measure the time it takes for the dye to disappear. A study that was conducted on cells of the upper-inner arms, a skin area previously shown to retain strength and resilience, showed the average cell transit time in young people 18 to 30 years old to be about twenty days. In contrast, skin cells in people 70 to 80 years old took thirty-seven days from origination to exfoliation. Further, there was no difference in the number of layers of skin cells in the two groups—the cells in both groups of people had the same journey to make. So skin cell renewal in elderly people takes almost twice the time it takes in young people.

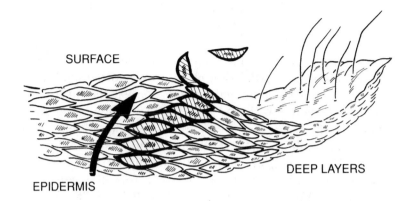

SURFACE

DEEP LAYERS

EPIDERMIS

Figure 12 The skin: Cells in transit. The human epidermis is a multi-layered system of cells constantly on the move—up. Each cell makes the journey (shown by the outlined cells) from the deepest layer to the surface, where it sheds. The life span of a skin cell ranges from about 20 days, in young people, to 37 days or more in old people. This is called "cell transit time." Skin is the largest organ of the body, weighing about 6 pounds and covering 3,000 square inches in an adult. Its thickness can vary from about one-fiftieth of an inch (eyelid) to one-third of an inch (palms and soles). It uses about a third of the body's circulating blood.

In early 1988, a report on tretinoin ointment received sensational media coverage. Researchers at The University of Michigan looked at the faces and forearms of thirty persons whose average age was 50, and found that after sixteen weeks of applying the ointment there was slight regression of sun-induced wrinkling and pigment discolorations. They also noted a potential benefit of tretinoin as therapy for skin cell abnormalities such as the nevus, actinic keratosis, and even melanoma, but it was the news about retarding wrinkling that caught the headlines. This illustrates our society's pre-dominant interest in the appearance of our skin rather than its health.

It is often said that if you want to guess a woman's age, look at the skin on the back of her hand. Skin is the external indicator of our age, and its texture, its wrinkles and lines, its thinning, and its loss of elasticity tell the tale, no matter how we try to disguise these changes. Losing extra pounds when we are young rather than later pays off because the skin, over the years, loses some of its capacity to contract. The result: sag marks for older dieters, especially on the arms and the buttocks. The stretching and retracting capacities of the skin become most evident to women during and after pregnancy, for abdominal skin must then stretch and retract prodigiously.

Skin very definitely ages at a rate corresponding directly to its exposure to sunlight. A recent study made at the University of Pennsylvania showed that skin ages at different rates on different parts of the body; exposed skin becomes wrinkled and covered skin ages more slowly. In the study in Pennsylvania, investigators looked at skin from different parts of the bodies of young and old people and they recorded the patterns of tiny wrinkles or furrows that they could see microscopically in the superficial, keratinous, top layer of skin. They found major differences between young and old skin in places such as the cheek and the dorsal sides of the hand and arm—places that are usually exposed. Young skin had a crisp, orderly geometric cell configuration. The scientists said the pattern resembled well-placed cobblestones or a cross-section of a honeycomb. The skin, though, on the other (older) hand, of people 65 to 80 years old did not show such an orderly pattern: Furrows were shallow and the cobblestone configurations were not to be seen. Most striking to the scientists was their finding that the skin of old people in parts of the body not exposed to the elements, parts such as the upper-inner arm, the abdomen, and the buttocks, was not much different from the young people's skin. In old skin from areas of the body that are normally covered, the scientists saw the same pattern of tightly packed cobblestones that they saw in young skin.

Manufacturers of "anti-aging" skin lotions promise that

by using their products, purchasers' skin will absorb collagen and elastin and, therefore, will look younger. Some of them go so far as to say that our skin, after we follow the instructions on the jars, will "be" younger. It must be admitted that most of us fall for these promises, even when science has repeatedly published findings that collagen and elastin cannot be absorbed by the body. They are proteins made only inside the human body and they work only in the particular body where they are made. In other words, they come not from a jar but from within. Further, our proteins are unique to us; they are highly personal products. Collagen is the protein found throughout the body, not just in the skin, that quite literally holds us together. It forms a system of cables giving the skin its strength so that when we pull on it it does not become detached. Elastin is another protein intermingled with collagen and it adds the property of elasticity to the skin. We can pinch the skin at our waists, as the television commercials show, and it will stretch and return to its shape like a rubber band. Collagen and elastin are responsible. Why do we lose some of this capacity as we age?

Japanese scientists have described a process called cross-linking that they observed in aging collagen molecules. They found that collagen in infants forms fairly short, separate cables of molecules. When they looked at the collagen in people of advancing years, though, they saw that the cables were longer and were often joined to other cables. Collagen molecules tend to join others to form even longer cables and then to cross-link to other cables. An explanation for this, offers the Japanese study, lies in the action of free radicals—stray molecules that can wedge between two cables (say, at a point where two labile or easily joined amino acids wait) and cause the chemical reaction of binding of the cables. The cables attach to each other. Where skin is concerned, more is not better: Collagen, compounded by cross-linked cables, becomes stiff and our skin loses its youthful resilience.

Cross-linking does not occur merely in collagen in the skin but it happens everywhere in the body. Examples are the

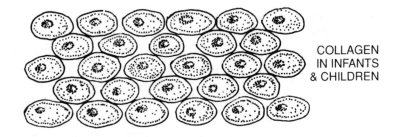

COLLAGEN
IN INFANTS
& CHILDREN

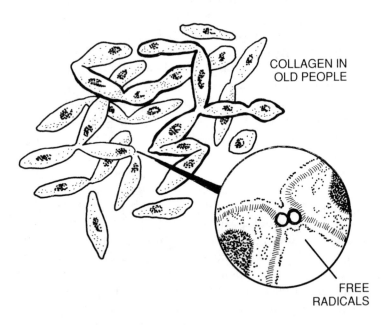

COLLAGEN IN
OLD PEOPLE

FREE
RADICALS

Figure 13 Collagen cross-linking: Molecules of collagen in the skin of very young people are more or less the same size (top drawing) and form orderly cables which produce a cobblestones pattern when seen microscopically. In contrast, the cables of collagen in old people (below) are disorderly, the molecules form irregular shapes, and the cables often "crosslink" to other cables, according to a recent study, through the binding of free radicals.

lens of the eye where the result of cross-linking is a cataract, and in the blood vessels where the result can be arteriosclerosis. Changes of age in the blood vessels directly affect the skin, since skin relies on oxygen-rich blood for its cell renewal. Collagen also holds veins and arteries together, and skin depends on the blood vessels to bring oxygen to it, so it is a delicately cross-linked biological setup.

As we age, we notice that cuts, scrapes, and bruises take a little longer to heal. This should be no cause for alarm—wound healing takes longer when cell renewal time is a longer process. Research into the skin's role in the body's immune defense provides fascinating new discoveries. Our skin, of course, as our interface with the world, acts as our first line of defense—our protective shield. But recently it has been found that certain skin cells which produce keratin, the protein of the tough outer epidermal layer such as of fingernails, toenails, and of hair, are quite similar to epithelial cells in the thymus (the immune system's center for lymphocyte maturation).

Our nails grow more opaque and ridged as we age and they grow more slowly. Between the ages of 20 and 80 there is an almost forty percent drop in their growth rate.

Another research finding was that the increased cell renewal time in old people is not a gradual, progressive change, as most aging adjustments are. The investigators found that there was not much of a change in cell transit time until about age 50 when cell renewal time changed profoundly. Skin cell replenishment remained fairly constant up to age 50, at which time it began to drop. Other changes include a reduction of melanocytes (pigment cells) which decrease almost 80 percent by age 65. Melanocytes gravitate toward the epidermis when we get a sun tan and their reduced numbers make it difficult for very old people to tan well. The sweat glands, tiny sacs in the skin, also diminish in number, leaving us with less capacity to cool off rapidly after a temperature rise when we are elderly. In general, our skin's water content drops somewhat as we grow older, along with a progressive dehydration of the body's tissues, and this change means the skin thins and sags because we have less subcutaneous fat.

Can these changes in wrinkling, cross-linking of collagen, cell renewal time, melanocytes, and water content be altered? Modern science has not yet found a way, and that is because the biological mechanisms that control these cell functions are basically not known. We will not have a way to change the rate of our skin's aging until we have some understanding about how the complex human coating develops and renews—much more understanding than we currently have about cross-linking and cell transit time.

Meanwhile, the people in the business of skin care have scientists on their payrolls and they, too, say that creams with vitamin E or estrogens contain rejuvenative miracles. But this is a science with selling products as its objective—there is no evidence that any of these claims are correct. Lotions and potions may clean our skin and some creams may soften it or supplement some natural skin oils that are not secreted as much when we are old, but for any other purpose they are worthless.

There is plenty of evidence showing that we can keep our skin healthy in ways that do not cost a lot of money. One important thing to do is to minimize exposure to direct sunlight. Another is to keep the skin clean by vigorously massaging it with a favorite soap. Why? Because cleaning and massaging keep the pores and pathways open for oxygen, the essential catalyst for renewal. We can exercise the skin—if only by standing in front of a mirror to see how many funny faces we can make. Why? Because by exercising the muscles we keep good, healthy connective tissue and muscle-skin attachment sites.

And why is jogging and other vigorous exercise good for the skin? A jogger bounces, causing the skin all over the body to jiggle, which stimulates the skin to tone up, again, by enhancing the attachments of skin to the underlying connective tissues and to muscle. Thus, skin is not loose but, rather, it clings to its attachments and it will stay taut and resilient.

Predisposition to Gray?

The control of all hair growth is probably hormonal. Teenaged boys are elated when, at puberty, there is a surge of androgens in their bodies and they begin to grow facial and other sexual hair. But all of our hair growth and hair loss throughout life is modulated by our hormones which are, again, like proteins, very personal. So hair is directed by glands—the thyroid, adrenal, gonadal, hypothalamus, and the pituitary. Since hormonal control lies ultimately in the brain, it is fairly safe to assume that it is there where hair changes are scheduled.

There are as many different changes, with age, in the color and pattern of human hair as there are human beings. We all turn gray and we are all becoming bald at our own pace. What is important for each of us is our own rate at which these changes occur. Besides the personal variability of hair changes, there are distinct racial differences which predispose hair pattern and loss. To be Caucasian is to have the greatest predisposition to graying and to becoming bald. People with a northern European ancestry have the greatest variety of possible hair color—black, brown, red, blond— and all shades of each, but their hair turns gray sooner than any other people's. Caucasian males become bald more frequently and at earlier ages than any other people do. When Oriental and black people's hair turns gray, it does so at a later age, sometimes not at all, and the same is true of hair loss. Far fewer Oriental and black men than Caucasians go bald, and when they do, it is at a later age. No one knows for sure why hair changes are so different among the races but genetics and, perhaps, dietary and environmental factors are instrumental.

What can these racial differences t   is about aging and

hair? Changes in hair, like proteins, are very personal matters. We each have a genetic predisposition to go gray at a certain time, whether we are male or female, and hair loss rates, too, are family-related. Some men are genetically predisposed to start to go bald, or more correctly, start to go down the road of their distinctive male pattern baldness at quite early ages; indeed, it often is apparent when they are in their twenties. For Caucasians that is early, but it happens often enough that it is not uncommon. What is uncommon is for many men to ever go completely bald. Actually, we are all losing hair all the time, moving toward a more or less typical pattern of baldness on top with a semi-circle of remaining hair from ear to ear. Women lose hair just as men do, but at slower rates. Very old women usually have very thin white hair.

Physically, what is happening to our hair as we age? Some facts are known. Graying, for example, is related to melanocytes, cells that make the pigment that gives our hair its distinctive color (as they do also in skin). In aging, there is a progressive loss of our numbers of melanocytes and a loss in the productivity of our remaining melanocytes. Without any pigment at all, that is to say, without functioning melanocytes, hair would appear to be white (as is the case with albinos). The process of graying is very gradual and it occurs at different rates in different areas of the body. A man's mustache and beard will probably turn gray before his scalp hair does. And when the scalp hair starts to turn gray, it usually begins at the temples.

Some facts about baldness and aging are also known. Hair, for example, does not simply fall out. Hair follicles go through a transition from making the large hair characteristic of the scalp to making a tiny, white hair called a vellus. A close inspection of a bald man's scalp reveals a covering of tiny, short, fuzzy, white or almost clear hair. Baldness rarely happens overnight, but thinning occurs in everyone gradually, each hair follicle less thick by about one-third when we are elderly. By age 70, our hair has become as fine as it was when we were babies.

Our Most Durable Parts

With our teeth, we are blessed with eating instruments that will last far longer than the rest of us—if we take care of them. A good illustration of the durability of our teeth has recently come to light with the exhumation of several hundred skeletons at Herculaneum, a seaport in Italy which, along with Pompeii, was devastated by the eruption of Vesuvius in A.D. 79. Most of the skeletons, buried for almost two thousand years, have beautifully-preserved teeth—still white and shiny, free of cavities. Historians and archeologists tell us the ancient Romans used no sugar in their diet. What they had problems with, though, like we do, was periodontal disease. Why? They had no dental floss.

Our teeth are the most durable of our body parts. Mother Nature designed them to last about two hundred years in the absence of preservation in volcanic ash. If we never ate sucrose and never developed gum disease, our teeth would serve us all our days. The loss of our teeth is a good example of the environmental theory of aging; it is the wear and tear of modern eating habits that ages them. All of our technological know-how goes into making substitutes for natural enamel, but neither gold nor space-age plastics are completely satisfactory substitutes for the real thing; teeth yellow from age are better than no teeth at all.

Good oral health is a prerequisite for good nourishment. The loss of our teeth means diet restrictions and alterations often resulting in poor nutrition. It is another vicious circle: Poor nutrition accelerates problems of the mouth such as tooth decay, jawbone loss, and delays in healing. It is amazing how many people believe that the natural life cycle progression is to lose one's teeth and get dentures. That is far from the truth. And dentures do not work as well as your own teeth. A dentist's decision to pull out a set of teeth should always be backed by a second—and even a third—opinion.

Nowadays, periodontal disease is the primary reason we lose our teeth as we grow old. As adults, we are beyond the "cavity-prone years." The reason is that most of the likely spots for caries, if you are caries-prone, are already filled with silver or gold. Statistics show that periodontal disease is truly epidemic: Almost seventy-five percent of us are victims of it between the ages of 18 and 80. For the elderly, the situation is more grim. Periodontal disease hits ninety percent of people over 65. We simply do not listen to our dentists. They scold us and lecture us about cleaning our teeth, flossing, and exercising tooth support structures by chewing. It seems, however, that they reach only about twenty-five percent of the population.

Gum disease is the result of a film on our teeth called plaque. Serious, regular brushing and flossing helps keep plaque off the surface of teeth, but it takes a dentist or a dental hygienist to keep it from spreading under the gingiva—the gum covering the jawbone and the roots of our teeth. When the plaque pushes the gingiva away from the teeth, bacteria can enter and cause infection. Then chronic inflammation causes the bone and ligaments that anchor the teeth to recede so the teeth, no longer held in place, start to rock excessively in their sockets. When this happens, the tooth is lost. You cannot cap or crown an unhealthy tooth— one that has substantially lost its support. You have to remove it. The ensuing infection can be a severe one causing bacteremia, a systemic disease.

People who cannot afford the high cost of dental care seem fated to develop periodontal disease. Most medical insurance excludes dental hygiene; Medicare does not cover it. The recent trend in large corporations to include dental insurance with medical benefits for employees is a good sign. Placing a crown on a decayed tooth can cost several hundred

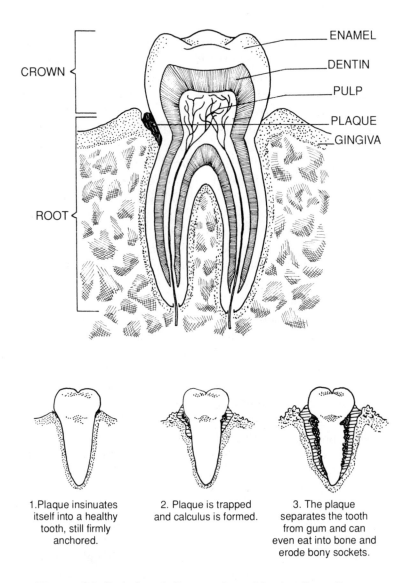

CROWN {

ENAMEL

DENTIN

PULP

PLAQUE

GINGIVA

ROOT {

1. Plaque insinuates itself into a healthy tooth, still firmly anchored.

2. Plaque is trapped and calculus is formed.

3. The plaque separates the tooth from gum and can even eat into bone and erode bony sockets.

Figure 14 Periodontal disease: An epidemic. Gum disease affects 75% of Americans over age 18, and 90% over age 65. Unremoved plaque can eventually push the gingiva away from the teeth, allowing bacteria to cause infection which destroys ligaments and bone that normally hold the teeth in place.

dollars these days; replacing a set of teeth lost to periodontal disease costs thousands. Dentists can afford to scold us.

Under the enamel of teeth is dentin, transparent living tissue. And under that, in the center of the tooth, is dental pulp, filled with nerves and blood vessels. Dental pulp diminishes as we age, through cell loss, dehydration, and vascular disease. Over the years, the gingiva loses keratin, the same protein coating which in other forms protects hair, skin, and fingernails. Aging, therefore, increases the possibility of inflammation of the gums—especially if there is bleeding, because the tissue is thin and susceptible to trauma. The periodontal ligament, a cushion between the teeth and their bone sockets, allows us to chew without cracking the teeth at their base. Arteriosclerosis accompanies aging and can impede some of the circulation needed to maintain the ligament's resiliency.

Arthritis, another condition often accompanying aging, can affect the jaw—particularly the temporomandibular joint which we use in chewing. If it hurts to chew, we stop chewing and the onset of periodontal disease is hastened. In many sick elderly people, "cotton mouth" (salivary gland disfunction) affects nutrition, since saliva is a mixture of proteins which begin the digestive process. It is also true that foods just do not taste right when the salivary gland is not working. Cancer often stops secretions of saliva, as do chemotherapy and radiation treatments for cancer. Saliva substitutes are available and they help.

Chewing is what our teeth were designed to do; it keeps them healthy. Exercising our teeth on anything chewy—from granola to spare ribs—will help their longevity. The regular exercise of chewing and the regular use of dental floss and a tooth brush are not expensive, and they are our best insurance.

A memorable scene in the Broadway musical play *A Little Night Music* by Stephen Sondheim and Hugh Wheeler occurs when an elderly grande dame character laments the losses in her life. It is unfortunate, she says, lecturing her granddaughter, to lose over the years a husband, two lovers, and a fortune. But to lose one's teeth, she declares, is nothing short of a catastrophe.

Chapter 8

Exercise and the Muscular System

Did President Kennedy conceive that his comments on physical fitness would inspire the exercise revolution we are witnessing today? He asked Americans to forgo their sedentary hours of television watching in favor of exercising the body and the mind. If he were around today, he would no doubt be dismayed to learn that television takes up, on the average, more hours of our day than it did in 1960. At the same time, there can be no doubt that he would rejoice to see the crowded "health spas" of the 1980's, the aerobics classes broadcast on television, the joggers of all ages running singly along the neighborhood streets or by the thousands in spectacular marathons, the helmeted bicyclists commuting to work with briefcases strapped behind them, and the bookstores brimming with exercise manuals and videos. President Kennedy was also a reader and there is no doubt that he would be avidly attuned to today's research in exercise and aging. Study after study reveals that life is indeed prolonged when regular exercise forms a part of the daily routine. Recent findings make it clear that exercise can slow down—even halt—our age-related rises in cholesterol and insulin blood levels, our loss of bone mineral, and our decreased cardiovascular function.

The fountain of health can flow through the aging years just as it flows through our youth. To help maintain the flow, we need to make habit-forming adjustments which benefit us first by making us feel youthful, and second, by making us keep a healthy-looking appearance. The two most important habits that do more to guarantee good health and good appearance than anything else are regular, balanced nutrition and regular exercise. A regimen of exercise is, of course, very personal. Some people walk, some people lift weights, some people join aerobics classes. Any type of exercise is muscular movement that works through some intriguing biological mechanisms.

Evidence is accumulating, hard scientific evidence that regular exercise is good for us no matter how old we are. Many people take up an exercise program only to drop it after a day or two. How boring, they say. The secret to a successful exercise program is to choose a type of exercise that you will enjoy doing. If it is drudgery, you won't do it FOR THE REST OF YOUR LIFE.

A fundamental question our researchers are asking: Does a person become sedentary because the physical changes of age force him to slow down (or even halt) most activity? Does the wear and tear, over the years, of a physically active life make us weak in old age? Or is it the other way around? Can it be that sedentary habits prematurely age us? Are we victims of a preconceived notion that older people cannot exercise? A maxim of biological evolution is "Use it or lose it." It is well-known that immobility causes bone loss and longitudinal research studies attest to an increased mortality from cardiovascular disease in sedentary people. So the question provokes our attention: Do our muscles lose their strength because we fail to use them? Is it inactivity of body and mind that leads to reduced physical and mental strength?

Perhaps the most noticeable change that comes with aging (aside from graying and wrinkling) is the reduced amount of time we spend in physical exercise. A boy and girl in their early teens are likely to pass two hours daily, after school, in vigorous sports like basketball. When they are 20, though, chances are they will devote only two or three hours a week to a sport, an exhausting tennis match on Saturday morning. By the age of 30, they are busy planning a ski trip or a weekend of hiking—their exercise for the month—unless pushing the baby-stroller consumes all their recreation time. Their forties and fifties? Well, they will be good sports and huff and puff their way through a family tag football game at the Fourth of July picnic. Eating and drinking is more enjoyable, though. And by 70, for too many people, walking down the street to their favorite park bench is a fatiguing, if festive, outing.

Not many research studies have been made which record time spent in exercise by age groups. In the early Seventies, one such study reported that about thirty percent of boys and girls 14 years old spent more than three hours a week playing vigorously. But for people 65 years old the figure was a mere three percent. There is hope, of course. Things have started to change dramatically in very recent years, as sales of bicycles, roller skates, sweat clothing, and health club memberships attest. But the physical fitness devotees of the Eighties are mostly people under the age of 40.

Why don't middleaged and elderly people exercise more? It is partly, and undeniably, due to a traditional notion that we should act our age, whatever that is. Our culture tells us that roller skates are for young people and that park benches are for old people. Period. That is the way it is. Just in the last century a myth in our society held it that exercise was bad for the human body. Physical activity damaged the body, according to accepted thought, and it decreased longevity. It takes decades to adjust social conditioning away from myths such as that. But aging and reduced physical strength involve more than social conditioning. We and other animals experience a true change in physical capacity as we age. We cannot be champion hurdlers in our sixties nor can we hope to break Olympic endurance records even in our thirties. This reality of aging, however, hardly means we must become sedentary. The active elders of the Soviet state of Georgia, along with the spry, octogenarian mountain climbers of Pakistan and Ecuador, demonstrate for us the benefits of regular, routine exercise. No one has told them at a certain age they should stop tilling and harvesting and toting. They do not have park benches. Well, perhaps a rock or two along the hike where they can catch their breath.

Pumping Ions: How Hormones and Calcium Stimulate Muscles

Brain and brawn work together, the muscles acting when they are stimulated by the brain. The reason a stroke victim may become paralyzed is not because his muscles are harmed directly, but because of brain or nerve death and damage, resulting in a lack of muscle stimulation and, often, muscle atrophy. The athlete's skills are a combination of muscular tone and coordination, or movements, and mental decisions, or intentions. Mere brawn is nothing without a brain directing it. And the brain is useless without a healthy body to do its bidding.

There are other connections, too, between the nervous system and the muscular system. The brain's neural tissue and the tissue of muscles share a characteristic with stem cells: Stem cells and muscle cells are finite in number. If lost, they cannot be replaced. We are born with just so many muscles, so many cells, and that's it. We cannot gain new muscles by working out every day at the gym, no matter how long or how vigorously. What strenuous exercise does for us is to increase the size of the muscles we are born with. We can change the shape and size of our muscles, but not the number of cells composing them.

Muscle cells are stimulated into movement by the same sort of chemistry that connects nerve cells. Messages from the brain (or impulses) travel down the nerve cells like electricity travels along wires. The class of hormones called neurotransmitters bridge the gaps (or synapses) between nerve cells, carrying the impulses from one nerve to the next. It is also the neurotransmitters that carry the impulses from the nerve cells to the muscle cells. The hormones are molecules which bind to the muscle cells' membranes, thus delivering the impulse.

What happens next is a marvel of Mother Nature's biological engineering. How does the impulse translate the brain's thought or reflex into muscular movement? What happens, after the impulse arrives, to cause contraction of muscle cells? When the neurotransmitter binds to the membrane of the muscle cell it stimulates enzymes which, in turn, act upon certain molecules on the surface of the muscle cells. These molecules can be called "doughnut molecules"—they have holes which the enzymes cause to open. When they open, the doughnut molecules allow calcium, and only calcium, to enter or leave the muscle cells. The phrase weightlifters use, "pumping iron," really should be changed to "pumping ions," for technically, their efforts result in the pumping of calcium ions in and out of their muscles. The molecules of calcium entering the muscles are electrically charged. When they are inside the muscle cells, they act as little bridges for two proteins, myosin and actin, to contact each other and to contract the muscle cells.

A muscle cell is actually a long fiber with many nuclei. At one time in our evolutionary history, large numbers of individual cells joined to form long networks of cells, thus pooling their strength. A muscle is made of millions of these cells that are arranged like long tubes with the ability to shorten and lengthen themselves. And that is all muscles do—shorten and lengthen. The presence or absence of calcium is what makes them do it. All our movements are the result of contractions and extensions of our long muscle cells. The basic physiology of bending a finger is not different from tossing a javelin to a world record, except the latter requires the coordination of many more muscles. Some muscles are called extensors and some are called flexors because of their respective working positions at various bone joints. But they both enable movement by getting shorter or by getting longer.

Muscles come in three general types: visceral, cardiac,

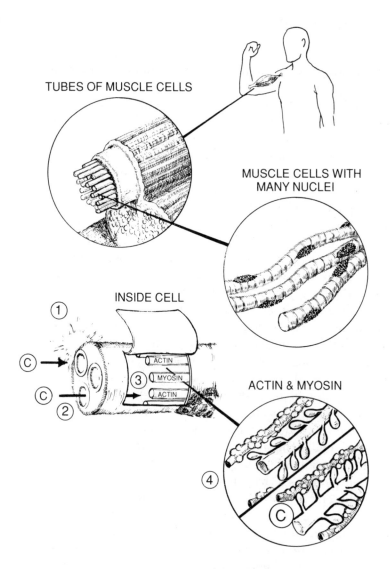

TUBES OF MUSCLE CELLS

MUSCLE CELLS WITH MANY NUCLEI

INSIDE CELL

ACTIN
MYOSIN
ACTIN

ACTIN & MYOSIN

Figure 15 How the muscles work: When a nerve impulse stimulates the muscle cell membrane (1), special "doughnut" molecules open to allow calcium (C) to enter (2). The calcium acts as a bridge for the filaments of myosin and actin (3), contractile proteins, to stretch and retract by a mechanism resembling paddles on a canoe (4).

and skeletal. Visceral muscles line the organs which have hollow cavities, such as the esophagus and the intestine. They contract and, in so doing, push food and waste along various tracts—digestive, gastrointestinal, urinary, and reproductive. Menstrual cramps are a manifestation of the slow, rhythmic contraction of visceral muscles. Cardiac muscles contract (or beat) to force blood in and out of the heart when they are stimulated by impulse-conducting cells. The nervous system actually does not initiate heart contractions but it regulates them. Skeletal muscle, the type of muscle we see, makes up the body's form and gives us our mobility and capacity for holding and lifting objects. They require nerve impulses, a biological mechanism called innervation, to function. They connect bones to each other at their ends, tendons, which are made of connective tissue.

Myosin and actin are called the contractile proteins and a tubular muscle cell consists of alternating filaments of them. One of them, myosin, comes with structures extending out from it like paddles on a canoe. When calcium comes into the cell, these paddles extend across to the actin and they stroke against the filament of actin, pushing just like paddles push against water to make a canoe move. At each end of the muscle tube the paddles pull the actin toward the center of the muscle cell. The millions of individual muscle cells contract, shortening the muscle that they form.

When the muscle has contracted, as originally planned by the brain and relayed through the nerve impulse, another impulse travels to the muscle cell membrane, resulting in flushing the calcium back out through the doughnut molecules. With no calcium to step on, the myosin paddles lose contact with the actin filament which slides back to its resting length; the muscle relaxes.

Detailed muscle physiology has taught us an important lesson about calcium. Without calcium the muscles cannot work. If a person's calcium stores in the bloodstream are deficient, his brain, not to be deterred, knows where to find it. To get muscular movement, the brain will extract calcium from the bones where it lies in great concentrations, and, for many aging people, decalcification of the bones results in osteoporosis. A calcium imbalance also causes painful chronic spasms in the abdominal muscles which is why people with osteoporosis often become pulled forward at the shoulders. If their vertebrae collapse, they become stoop-shouldered. Cramps and "charley horses" are other results of calcium imbalances when muscles contract but fail to relax. They can also be results of nerve signal misfiring or of a lack of blood supply to the muscles.

Why are we subject to cramps if we exercise strenuously just after eating? A large quantity of blood has just been diverted to the stomach to assist it in digestion. For the skeletal muscles of the body, the availability of blood, with its oxygen supplies, is temporarily reduced. That is also the reason why we are sleepy after a big meal. Our muscles do not have the oxygen they need for energy.

Calcium triggers muscle contraction and oxygen fuels it so movement can continue. The cells' energy factories, the mitochondria, "burn" oxygen to create adenosine triphosphate (ATP). It is the energy of ATP which provides the contractile proteins, myosin and actin, with the capacity to continue their work. Much of our physical effort, though, requires more energy faster than it can be converted from the amount of oxygen available in the bloodstream. And that is the difference in the terms aerobic and anaerobic.

Muscle contractions held to a pace not exceeding the amount of energy converted from available oxygen are aerobic contractions. Aerobic exercises include walking, dancing, jogging, swimming, bicycling, calisthenics, and the like. Rhythmic breathing is an important element of aerobic exercises; as oxygen is burned to make energy to keep the muscles going, more oxygen is inhaled for replenishment. People who are serious about "aerobics" keep a close watch on their pulse rate because they do not want to pass the point when more oxygen is required than is supplied—the maximum pulse rate. As a general rule, a person's maximum pulse rate is seventy-five percent of the number 220, minus his age.

Soreness and pain result from prolonged physical effort exceeding the body's oxygen-burning capacity. That is anaerobic effort, since the muscles' energy must come from a source other than oxygen. In strenuous effort such as holding a heavy object or in sustained exercise requiring more than usual energy, the mitochondria must look to glycogen, the sugar from carbohydrate stored in the muscles. It is burned to make heavy-duty fuel to run the contractile proteins. Our anaerobic effort is limited at any age. The conversion of glycogen to energy creates a by-product of lactic acid in the muscles. This acid buildup, in turn, inhibits the myosin-actin contraction process, leaving the muscles sore and exhausted.

Taking Steps to Good Health

A hopeful, positive attitude is the first requirement for active later years. Can we really be hopeful about staying healthy and active? Yes, we can, but it takes more than hope. We should look at just what the changes are that are taking place in our muscular system as we age. Then we can take steps— literally—for minimizing the effects of those changes.

Muscle cell loss does not usually occur until very late in a person's life and then, usually, it is due to disease or disuse. But we lose strength and efficiency in our muscles as we age. There are several reasons: first, some lean mass in the muscles is inevitably lost and replaced by fat and connective (scar) tissue. That means our oxygen stores are reduced so the muscles must resort to anaerobic energy. Much physical effort which can be handled aerobically when we are young, in other words, becomes an anaerobic task—a potentially more fatiguing effort—when we are older.

Second, the contractile proteins, myosin and actin, may lose some of their function along with a loss of cells involved in the enzymatic binding and stimulating functions. Some of the muscle tube cells, therefore, do not contract, so overall strength is reduced. It is like a ten-man rowboat crewed by eight or nine rowers.

Third, a combination of things may happen: Nervous system adjustments of age obviously affect muscles' ability to react, as does the higher proportion of subcutaneous fat in our aging bodies which makes heat exchange more difficult. Heating and cooling are necessary for muscles to maintain their efficiency. Being overweight compounds the situation.

Fourth, stiffening of the joints is common in older people, making mobility more difficult. Inactivity results in a loss of muscle fiber which is replaced by connective tissue and then the muscles tend to become stiffer, and to tense, relax, and heal more slowly.

Fifth, balance is a problem for many oldsters, too, and it is believed that development of arteriosclerosis in the blood vessels of the ear is responsible.

The main reason we experience downward adjustments in muscular efficiency as we grow older is reduced oxygen consumption. Our blood can carry just as much oxygen when we are old as when we are young. On the other hand, an old person's lungs cannot get oxygen into the blood as quickly as they used to. The muscles operating the lungs weaken and other tissues of the chest cage stiffen so the lungs cannot expand quite so much. And the older heart cannot pump it as fast as it used to. Our "vital capacity," the maximum amount of air that can be inhaled, reduces when we age. The lung's functional change is due to cell loss, the loss of alveolar sacs, the loss of cilia, (the wavy, hair-like structures which clear mucus away), and a certain amount of loss of elasticity of the lung tissue. But our lungs were designed with such a great reserve capacity that the normal functional changes of age barely impede our breathing. And research has shown that exercise that forces our lungs to work hard will improve their functional performance. Along with a reduced heart rate, though, aging means that oxygen is not available to the muscles as quickly as it once was. So we may still flex our

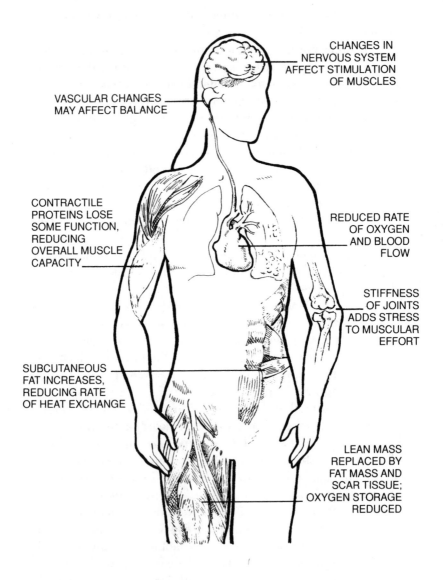

CHANGES IN
NERVOUS SYSTEM
AFFECT STIMULATION
OF MUSCLES

VASCULAR CHANGES
MAY AFFECT BALANCE

CONTRACTILE
PROTEINS LOSE
SOME FUNCTION,
REDUCING
OVERALL MUSCLE
CAPACITY

REDUCED RATE
OF OXYGEN
AND BLOOD
FLOW

STIFFNESS
OF JOINTS
ADDS STRESS
TO MUSCULAR
EFFORT

SUBCUTANEOUS
FAT INCREASES,
REDUCING RATE
OF HEAT EXCHANGE

LEAN MASS
REPLACED BY
FAT MASS AND
SCAR TISSUE;
OXYGEN STORAGE
REDUCED

Figure 16 The changing muscular system

muscles when we are old, albeit not so rapidly as when we are young.

If other cardiovascular problems exist in an aging person, say, hardening or thickening of the arteries, delivery of oxygen to the muscles is impeded even more than the normal adjustment. Quickly exhausting their aerobic energy, the muscles must then switch to the more taxing anaerobic process—using up ATP stores and manufacturing lactic acid. But an old person who exercises regularly will condition himself to minimize the effects of these changes.

Use It or Lose It

This chapter began by asking some questions: Is the loss of physical strength and endurance an inevitable corollary of the aging process? Is the loss due, or partly due, to a voluntary decrease in physical activity? By succumbing to sedentary ways are we causing our muscles to atrophy? Do we, in fact, lose our muscles when we do not use them?

The answers coming from research efforts may not yet be complete but they provide plenty of good reasons for our being hopeful.

Muscular movement is something we are not born knowing, but something we must learn. We teach our muscles their movements and their coordination of movements. As babies we start by crawling, then we toddle, then we walk. During those early months we are educating our muscles while they are growing. Movements are not instinctive; we learn by trial and error. Strenuous use of muscles in our youth causes them to grow large but not using muscles creates the opposite effect. For example, when we break an arm and cast it in plaster our arm muscles shrink because we are not using those muscles; when the cast comes off, it is our use of the muscles that restores their tone. Stroke patients who have lost nerves which carry impulses to certain muscles must go through the same process of reeducation of muscular movement, called rehabilitation. During the period before the nerves regenerate, the affected muscles atrophy because they are not being used. The muscles must learn anew to contract and the time it takes for their reeducation is in proportion to the length of time they are out of use. The exercises used in rehabilitation stimulate the muscles to contract and relax, thus maintaining their size and capacity.

Research has found that elderly people benefit from physical exercise just as young people do, if not as quickly. Researcher Herbert DeVries has reported that after a forty-two week exercise program for men in their seventies and eighties that was conducted by the University of Southern California, some stereotypes about old people and physical activity were thrown by the wayside. The exercise program clearly increased the strength and flexibility of the old men and DeVries found a twenty-nine percent improvement in oxygen consumption per heart beat. Physical training in young people rarely yields better results than that. An improvement of twenty percent was recorded in maximum breathing capacity. That means the old men, after ten months of regular exercise, could consume twenty percent more oxygen and, presumably, remain vigorously active twenty percent longer than before they started the program.

The exercise program the old men pursued consisted of the jog-walk—jogging a short distance and then walking the same distance, gradually increasing the jog portions. Swimming proved to be a good exercise for people with stiffness in knees, feet, and ankles. And elderly non-swimmers learned to swim just as easily as non-swimming college students do. Stretching exercises were used to alleviate muscle soreness. Calisthenics and yoga exercises helped build endurance. Joint mobility, which is often prone to stiffness in the elderly, improved with weightlifting exercises, and balance exercises restored some of the men's declining sense of balance.

Rhythmic or isotonic exercises appeared to be preferable for old people to isometric or contraction-holding exercises which may push blood pressure up.

And finally, the old men who took part in the program found an additional benefit: Regular exercise caused a net loss of fat. This was true even though they made no change in their diets.

Another study, this one conducted at the University of California, Los Angeles, showed that life expectancy for both men and women could be increased by six or seven years if "yes" was the response to each of the following questions:

—Do you usually sleep seven or eight hours a day?

—Do you usually eat breakfast?

—Do you eat three meals regularly and pass up in-between meal snacks?

—Do you maintain normal body weight?

—Do you exercise regularly and vigorously?

—Do you drink little alcohol?

—Did you never smoke or did you stop smoking?

A test of this kind, of course, cannot predict the life expectancy of an individual; it is a statistical study showing "averages." It is the kind of test used by insurance companies, since it yields expectations for great numbers of people, not for individuals. Even as statistical tools, these studies are somewhat biased. People who take part in them (those persons who respond to advertising for such a study) do so because they are already health-minded people. Their health is, on the average, better than the health of people "picked off the street" and, needless to say, in our society we do not pick people off the street for research; we rely on volunteers.

There are two kinds of research studies for observing the

effects of exercise on aging. One kind, cross sectional studies, are those which use a mixture of young, middleaged, and elderly people and report the differences among them. The other kind of study, a longitudinal aging study, is one that follows the same group of individuals from their youth to their old age to observe the changes taking place. The longitudinal study which began in the 1950s at the National Institute on Aging in Baltimore is now yielding myth-shattering findings but also it has some inherent problems for data accuracy. It has consisted of people who are more health-conscious than their average peers, and when changes occur in their health, how can you be certain that what you are observing is aging or disease? Well, usually the changes caused by acute disease occur more rapidly than changes from aging. On the other hand, there are many diseases marked by long, slow onsets. Do such diseases accelerate the aging process? In these matters, it must be repeated that there are all shades of gray.

Other studies, perhaps more significant for learning the effects of exercise, have been made on the physical effects of bed-rest or inactivity and on the weightlessness and relative physical inactivity of astronauts while they are in space. Physical changes occur rapidly in astronauts and in inactive people of all ages. The changes are remarkably similar to the changes that accompany aging.

The sense of balance, the body's water level, and our red blood cell mass all decline somewhat with age. Prolonged bed rest and weightless space flights produce the same changes in people. A reduction of lymphocytes, the immune system's disease-fighting soldiers, occurs in astronauts, in sick, immobile people, and in the elderly. In the absence of gravity, astronauts have lost lean body mass and calcium. When there is no gravitational force, there is no resistance to normal muscular movements. In the case of the astronauts, the lack of gravity means inactive muscles; sick people do not use their muscles while they are in bed. However, exercise programs for persons in flight or in bed have reversed these changes in lean mass and calcium amounts.

There are some studies suggesting that age-related bone loss can be retarded by moderate, regular exercise. In some cases, in fact, exercise has resulted in an increase of bone density. When J. L. Aloia evaluated the effect that one hour of exercise three times a week for one year had on women four years after their menopause, he found that their total body calcium increased measurably. But the body calcium levels decreased in the control group composed of women who did not exercise. E. L. Smith and W. Reddan studied the effects of exercise on elderly nursing home patients and reported increased bone mineral content after a three year regimen of doing moderate exercises while sitting in chairs for thirty minutes three times a week.

Other researchers are finding that long periods of physical inactivity cause changes in the body's central nervous system, in our sleep patterns, and in our sensory capacities. These changes approximate the longterm changes of very old age.

Just as disease can accelerate the inevitable changes of aging, so apparently can inactivity. Just as a lack of the essential nutrients in our diet means we are not providing the fuels we need for healthy chemical reactions, so a lack of physical activity means we are not maintaining good blood flow to the muscles. It seems clear that by not using muscles we are only hastening their decline. A leading cause of death in very old people—those over 75—is pulmonary embolism, a blood clot lodged in the pulmonary arteries. Often, the blood clots in the legs because of their inactivity. Then, it dislodges and comes to rest where it may block blood flow to the heart or the lungs. These people need to move about—or at least to exercise their legs—to keep blood flowing so it will not clot.

The death of jogging advocate Jim Fixx in early 1985 led, briefly, to echoes of the nineteenth century myth that exercise endangers the body. But it was soon reported that Fixx was genetically predisposed to heart disease and there has even been a research study showing that people who habitually and vigorously exercise are at less risk of heart disease than those who do not. D. S. Siscovick interviewed the wives of 133 men who had died from primary cardiac arrest (a medical term for sudden death). He found that while the chances of death occurring while exercising was slightly elevated for everyone, for those who did not habitually exercise, the risk was greatly increased. Among the physically active men, though, the overall risk of cardiac arrest during and after exercise was only forty percent that of the sedentary men. Other research done with laboratory dogs, pigs, and rats has proven that exercise stimulates the development of coronary collateral vessels, which, of course, reduce one's chances of sudden death following a heart attack. Finally, regular exercise leads to more healthful balances of HDL and LDL, the high-density and low-density cholesterol matter in the bloodstream. LDL, it has been shown, leads to clogging of the arteries when it overshadows the level of HDL. But when a group of athletes who had stopped exercising were appraised in a study at Brown University, it was found that their LDL levels had increased and their HDL levels had gone down. On the other hand, a group of athletes who continued to exercise (and who ate twenty percent fewer calories during the study) showed the opposite results: Their HDL rose, while their LDL decreased.

The best forms of physical exercise are the ones that benefit the whole body—walking, jogging, swimming, bicycling—by promoting blood flow through the heart to the other muscles and to the organs. The best time to exercise? Daily. Regularly. Just as with a diet, an exercise regimen is not designed for a month or for six months or for a year. It is for THE REST OF YOUR LIFE.

Chapter 9

The Blood Vessels: Aging's Barometer

One muscle never rests—the heart. Its "lifeblood" is good circulatory flow. If the heart may harden from lack of emotional use, as the poets say, it can weaken and strain from unhealthy bloodflow, as the physicians and scientists say.

Heart disease is on the decline in the United States. However, it still is our "number one killer," causing as many deaths annually as all other causes put together. Coronary heart disease, manifested clinically primarily by myocardial infarction (heart attack) and angina pectoris (chest pain), remains the major cause of death in industrial societies—there are more than a million heart attacks and half a million deaths annually, just in the United States. Since the early 1960s, though, deaths from heart disease have been decreasing. During the first half of the century, cardiovascular disease steadily claimed more and more lives. Because of new medicine and better sanitation, people began, for the first time in history, to live long enough to lose cardiovascular integrity. It is also speculated that the reasons for the rise in heart disease included the new reliance on automobiles, for Henry Ford did more than mass-produce an inexpensive machine for moving the masses: He put an end to walking. The high-protein, high-fat diet of America's prosperity also surely played a part in the climbing frequency of heart disease. Dietary fat intake increased twenty-five percent in the United States between 1900 and 1970, and complex carbohydrate intake decreased twenty-five percent. On the other hand, we ate more sugar (a simple carbohydrate). The cigarette, which enjoyed a glamorous status in the Thirties and Forties (before its ill effects became known), played havoc with coronary heart disease statistics. It is quite logical, therefore, to speculate that the current decline in deaths from cardiovascular disease is due to our increasing interest in exercise and nutrition, and to our decreasing interest in tobacco. Still, it was reported in early 1985 by the Journal of the American Medical Association that one-fifth of all Americans are twenty percent overweight. Half of all Americans are hyperlipidemic—their diets and lack of exercise promoting too much fat and cholesterol. "Is this not malnourishment?" asked the journal's editorial writer. Other reports showed that about a quarter of the adult population continues to smoke.

New medical techniques and tools can speed up a flagging heart, can stabilize a fluttering one, and even replace one that has given up. We take drugs that open clogged arteries with more reliability than products we make for blocked drain pipes. Certainly a major force in the decline of heart disease deaths is emergency treatment—ironically made possible by the automobile. Paramedics arrive quickly in ambulances to assist after a myocardial infarction, and family members and neighbors have learned CPR (cardiopulmonary resuscitation) through a massive teaching project by the American Heart Association.

When physicians tell us that we are as old as our blood vessels, they are describing a universal aging change. Everyone's arteries stiffen from an early age; indeed, the blood vessels are aging's barometer, and the fact is hardly news. The curious Greeks of early history theorized causes for arterial blockage and Leonardo da Vinci wrote about the thickened, inelastic blood vessels of old people whose bodies he examined. The cardiovascular system simply was not designed to last as long, say, as the two hundred year enamel of our teeth; arteries and veins start losing their elasticity in a fraction of that time, and fatty and calcium deposits impede the flow of blood through the vessels from our early childhood days. The heart's muscles and the smooth muscles of the blood vessels, which contract to squeeze and push blood and oxygen to every part of the body, are subject to a loss of strength (just as our muscles) when oxygen and calcium supplies decrease.

Occupying center stage in the cardiovascular system is the heart, the muscular organ which collects oxygenated blood from the lungs and propels it to all the parts of the body. At the same time that it pumps this "new blood," it pumps the already circulated "tired" blood to the lungs for an over-haul—carbon dioxide is removed from the blood and new oxygen is added. Diastole is the heart's moment of relaxation when fresh blood from the lungs and depleted blood from the body fill the two atria. Nerve impulses regulate the swing of the atrial valves so that the blood spills into the ventricles. Another nerve impulse then controls systole (contraction of the ventricles), forcing the blood out and on its way through the vessels.

Blood vessels come in varying sizes—from arteries such as the aorta, through which quarts of blood flow in seconds, to veins no thicker than toothpicks, and to capillaries so small and narrow that the red blood cells must travel through them single file. The ancient Latin word "vas" and the result-ant prefix "vaso" continue to denote vessel in our language. Thus, drugs called vasodilators act to dilate or widen a narrowed blood vessel.

Arteries and veins are made of layers of cells—similarly to the skin, but with specialized function. Endothelial cells line the inside of the vessels, surrounded by a layer of smooth muscle cells which contract in a different way from other muscles. Their actions are to constrict and to expand the vessel, regulating flow and pressure. There are other muscle fibers similar to those of our limb and trunk muscles and the connective tissues, elastin and collagen, function also in the vessels' structure.

Not center stage, but taking supporting roles in the cardiovascular system, are the lungs, the liver, the kidneys, and the spleen. Like the lungs, these other organs service the blood in some way. The liver removes toxins from the blood and the kidneys purge it of uric acid, ammonia, water, and excess sodium, potassium, and calcium. The spleen is a rigorous filter. It has orifices so small that only red blood cells strong enough to hold their shape are able to squeeze through. The weak ones are not allowed to pass.

Responses to Stress

How does the cardiovascular system change with age? The changes are manifold and complex and so are the diseases of the system. In fact, it is often difficult to distinguish between the system's predictable aging changes and its inevitable diseases. It is often said by layman and by scientist alike that much heart disease is related to, or influenced by, aging changes.

Every physical effort we make requires an increased heartbeat rate. Our "resting" heart rate is our normal pulse of blood flow, but for physical effort such as walking or brushing our teeth, an increased rate of supplying blood and oxygen to the muscles is required. For experimental purposes, when groups of young adults and groups of old adults attempt various tests of physical effort such as pedalling laboratory bicycles, the studies show that a young person's heart rate increases more than the old person's. Physicians and scientists call this increased blood flow "response to stress," our body's way of accommodating physical work or effort. The old heart cannot pump as much blood as quickly as the young heart can. A healthy old person tires from physical exertion more quickly than a healthy young person does because cardiac reserve capacity in the young allows for a quadrupling of cardiac output, the volume of blood the heart pumps per beat. The trained athlete's cardiac output can increase six times when he calls upon all his powers, and, nice to know, an observed fact among elderly people who have continued to exercise regularly is their enhanced cardiac reserve.

In the typical human being, however, cardiac output decreases after about age 20 at a rate of almost one percent each year. This fall in output is thought to be mainly due to changes in our body size. A body whose muscles and organs have become smaller than they were requires less circulating blood. Many other observable changes in the heart affect its output: The wall of the left ventricle grows thicker by as much as twenty-five percent; the interior muscle layer, the endocardium, thickens a little with a buildup of connective tissue; the heart's valves grow thicker and more rigid due to the presence of more collagen and cross-linking (the same change so prominent in aging skin); the number and size of the heart's muscle fibers gradually reduce; and lipofuscin (a yellowish, ear wax-like cellular waste product) accumulates, thought to have the effect of impeding muscle contraction.

All this is not to say the heart of a healthy older person cannot pump as well as a young adult's heart. It can and does, for the strength and speed of heart contractions change little. The changes in cardiac output mean the older heart cannot provide its reserve capacity as quickly as it once did. The older person needs a little more time for homeostasis to adjust to physical exertion.

The heart's changing output is also due to the gradual and inevitable stiffening of the arteries, creating resistance to blood flow. On the average, pulse rate goes from a baby's 140 beats per minute to half that in a young adult. A young person's thoracic aorta, the largest artery we have, is so elastic it can expand three times its normal diameter when cardiac output rises in response to physical exertion such as running. As we approach age 80, though, the elasticity of the thoracic aorta will allow only about a fifty percent expansion. This affects the heart's output since the maximum blood flow through the coronary arteries (the vessels bringing blood and oxygen to the heart's muscles) may be reduced by one-third at

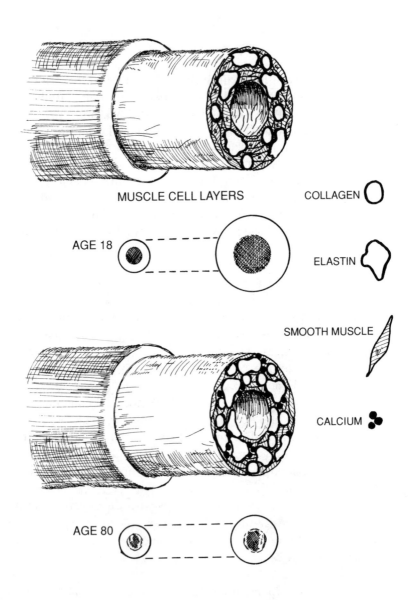

Figure 17 The aging aorta: The young vessel, depicted at the top, can expand to three times its normal size to accommodate increased blood flow. By age 80, shown below, the proportions of collagen and elastin have shifted, and calcium is present, so the aorta can expand by only 50%.

age 60. Just as in the skin, elastin decreases in the arteries, while collagen increases. What's more, a property of elastin is the attraction of calcium; so, as the arteries grow less elastic, they become more calcified too. Hardening of the arteries happens in all people and animals, a fact of aging, even though the aorta and other arteries stretch somewhat to compensate for the general stiffening. While young arteries expand to accommodate increased cardiac output, stretching is the vessels' way to adjust for their declining capacity to expand. The loss of elasticity of the aorta also contributes to the instability of the regulation of blood pressure that is so common in the elderly.

The aorta helps the heart by acting almost as a ventricle; it receives just-pumped blood and pulses right along with the heart to give the blood an extra push. Because the aorta stretches with age, it loses some of its capacity to contract and push the blood. This is true of the other arteries, but not of the veins, whose role of returning blood to the heart is more passive than the arteries' active role as expediters. When blood volume increases in an artery, at the same time the artery's capacity to expand has been reduced by stiffening; the blood's pressure against the arterial walls increases— hypertension. Normally, the brain senses this increased pressure and through nerve signals instructs the smooth muscles of the blood vessels to contract, pushing some of the blood, and shifting the volume to even out the pressure. So while hypertension is not nervousness, but rather, elevated blood pressure in the vessels, the nervous system does play a part; it serves to check and balance the blood's pressure against the vessel walls.

On the average, the resistance of the vessels to blood flow increases steadily over the years. Experimental studies show that the rate of the increased resistance is slightly more than one percent each year, the same rate as our decrease in cardiac output. This means the heart must work harder to pump blood to all the muscles and organs. Our bodies try to compensate not only through brain signals to ease the pressure, but also by making new capillaries, thus increasing vascularization—new passageways for blood to go where it is needed.

The kidneys assist blood flow by glomerular filtration, regulation of the sodium and other salts in the blood. Too much sodium in the blood means that blood volume increases because the concentration of salt must be maintained at a critical level. A high level of salt in the blood brings on thirst, so that more fluid will be added to the blood. As the kidneys age, they lose some of their glomeruli (the filters) and thus they cannot filter as rapidly as before. Some studies show that by age 90, a person's kidneys are functioning only half as well as they were at age 20. The kidneys are thickly vascularized so that blood and oxygen can easily reach the glomeruli. All these vessels of the kidneys are subject to stiffening and other forms of clogging, too, so blood volume in the kidneys is reduced with age. The reduced amount of blood means some glomeruli do not get oxygen so they starve and die.

As vessel resistance rises and kidney filtration falls, blood pressure becomes greater while the delivery of oxygen and other nutrients through the body becomes more of a task for the heart. When a physician measures a person's blood pressure, the two numbers he records (for example, 120/80, a so-called normal measurement) represent different types of pressure. To obtain them, the pressure in the cuff around the upper arm is increased so that the blood flow stops. The first number, systolic pressure, is the point on the gauge when the air pressure in the cuff is released and blood starts to flow again. It symbolizes the energy needed to hold back the blood flow. Because the left ventricle wall grows thicker as we age, systolic pressure increases by some fifteen percent. The second number, diastolic pressure, is a measure of the force of the resumed blood flow when the cuff is loosened and there is no resistance.

Not everyone has hypertension, of course, a disease more predominant in Western society than in other parts of the world. It is most frequent in Black people. Almost all studies show that if you have high blood pressure when you are young, you can expect it to increase as you age. On the other hand, if you start with low blood pressure, you can expect some increase as you age, but less than a person who has always had high blood pressure. And low blood pressure, hypotension, can present its own problems. The aging decrease in heart beat volume and the increase in the volume held by the stretched aorta can lead to hypotension. Not enough blood is circulating quickly enough. People with low blood pressure must be careful when they change positions, for example, when they stand or sit up suddenly from lying down. Their blood cannot move as quickly as they need it to. Changing position or exerting themselves abruptly can cause them to faint or, at the least, have a little dizziness or lightheadedness.

Several high risk factors are related to high blood pressure. Being overweight is very dangerous. Fat impedes expansion of the smooth muscles of the vessels and it impedes blood perfusion (the exchange of oxygen and nutrients), the principal reason blood circulates. It also increases the probability of formation of fatty deposits on the insides of the blood vessels. A diet high in salt is a high risk for high blood pressure patients because salt attracts fluid, increasing the blood's volume in aging vessels that are stiffening. Chronic stress, whether mental or physical, increases blood flow which meets resistance from less elastic older vessels. Blood pressure can be affected by the changing regulatory functions of the nervous system and the endocrine system. If secretions of the hormone aldosterone drop off as we age, salt content of the blood can go unregulated—especially when kidney filtration is also dropping. Nerve signals for contraction and expansion of the vessels' muscles may lose accuracy as we age. This is probably cigarette smoking's greatest threat to the cardiovascular system—smoking interferes with neurotransmitters, so they fail to deliver their impulse for muscle contraction and blood flow is impeded. Good news: The Baltimore Longitudinal Study on Aging reports that when middleaged or older people stop smoking, lung function returns to normal after eighteen to twenty-four months.

Regulation and compensation are biological processes. Changes in the body's way of doing things, its metabolism, are normally accompanied by compensations. When lung capacity drops due to loss of air sacs, we develop previously unused chest muscles to aid in using previously infrequently used areas of the lungs. We use the newly developed chest muscles for breathing. If the kidneys and the liver lose parts of their structures, new blood vessels develop to compensate for the decreased surface area for blood exchange. Changes in one of the body's systems are compensated for by adjustments in other systems—homeostasis. A good example is the nervous system's regulation of blood pressure. The loss of this regulation—the ability of one system to compensate for changes in other systems—is perhaps the hallmark of the aging process.

Arteriosclerosis or Atherosclerosis?

Arteriosclerosis is perhaps one of the best understood changes of age. Science can describe the reasons for the inevitable stiffening of our blood vessels, although atherosclerosis, a disease often confused with arteriosclerosis, retains pathogenic mystery. Not long ago, arteriosclerosis (hardening of the arteries) was an umbrella term embracing other heart and cardiovascular system conditions—myocardial infarction, atherosclerosis, coronary artery spasm, tachycardia (a fibrillating heart, the "flutters") and arrhythmias, and even hypertension. But research in the last couple of decades has shown that all of us have arteriosclerosis to some degree. Hardening or stiffening of the arteries is a part of aging, just as skin wrinkles and becomes thin and inelastic. The same aging processes that are occurring on the outside of our bodies are occurring on the inside. Not everyone, though, has heart attacks, hypertension, or serious atherosclerosis.

The blood vessels stiffen primarily because of changes in their structure as we age due to changes occurring in the cellular components of the vessels. A substantial amount of smooth muscle and the proteins elastin and collagen make up about a third of the weight of arteries, but over the years, collagen, the connective tissues appearing in other parts of the body in other forms, slowly predominates. Researchers say we have lost about a third of our arteries' elastin when we reach an advanced age. And they have shown that the connective collagen increases from about twenty percent of arterial weight in our twenties to more than twenty-five percent in our eighties. There is an increased tendency for collagen to become cross-linked, as it does in the skin, adding further to the stiffening of the vessels. It is a gradual aging change and, like everything human, the rate of the change is highly variable from person to person. Some researchers suggest that elastin loss is related to an accumulation of fats and cholesterol in the arteries. Others say that elastin molecules attract polysaccharides, or carbohydrates, which bind to them, altering their makeup so they lose their property of being elastic. Elastin binds to the mineral calcium, and so calcification takes place in arteries as it does in our joints.

A good way to accelerate arteriosclerosis is to overeat. Excess fats and carbohydrates in the bloodstream, by biological processes not thoroughly understood, hasten the stiffening process. Hypertension exacerbates the condition since the continual stretching of the vessels causes further loss of their elastic properties by simple wear and tear. Being male is to be more susceptible to arteriosclerosis than being female, a fact believed to be related to hormonal regulation. Not long ago, it was thought to have to do with stress, but years after women had entered the workplace in large numbers their expected rise in heart disease did not materialize. The old wives' tale that women are better equipped to handle stress than men may be true. It's their hormones. On the other hand, female heart disease due to cigarette smoking has shown a definite increase.

Chronic stress (in both sexes) leads to hypertension and therefore it can be said to accelerate arterial stiffening. Racial and geographic differences also affect the rate of arteriosclerosis. The most significant correlation is one we can do nothing about: growing old. Hardening of the arteries is a fact of everyone's life.

While arteriosclerosis is an aging change seen in all people, atherosclerosis is a disease and does not occur in everyone. Atherosclerosis is deadly; it blocks the flow of blood and can therefore kill us with hardly any warning. When antibiotics tamed infectious diseases and sanitation was improved early in this century, many people began to live long enough to become victims of atherosclerosis, although in some the disease process starts at a very young age. In its most advanced forms, it blocks blood flow to any organ but its most serious consequences affect the heart or the brain. The reason we die from atherosclerosis is organ failure—the artery to that organ did not deliver blood and oxygen. We have strokes from atherosclerosis because blood-carried oxygen is blocked from a portion of the brain. If blood is cut off from any part of the body, that part starves and dies.

Fatty deposits or plaques in the blood vessels (called atheromas) accumulate most frequently at points where the blood vessel splits in two. The most common arteries where they form are the coronary arteries and the aorta. But the rate of their formation varies from person to person. In childhood, these deposits may be tiny lesions in the vessels. They are small collections of fats and cholesterol in the smooth muscle tissue. As we age, the deposits grow in size and by the time we are adults, they are called plaques—atherosclerotic plaques. They are like scars then and are made of more than fat and cholesterol; they have accumulated collagen, sugars, their own capillaries, white blood cells, and, usually, calcium. In effect, they are localized bulges of accelerated hardening; calcification replaces elasticity, contributing to high blood pressure and to general arteriosclerosis.

High Density Lipoproteins and Low Density Lipoproteins

Explanations for the genesis of atheromas are still more in the realm of theory than of fact. Because people have different DNA-coded instructions for producing proteins, we all have different quantities of specific enzymes that break down molecules of fats in our food. And some studies seem to show there is a decrease in this enzymatic capacity as we age, so that more fats are left to circulate in the blood vessels.

Michael Brown and Joseph Goldstein, professors of medicine and genetics at the University of Texas Health Science Center at Dallas, recently observed and described a biological mechanism in the body for controlling quantities of cholesterol—a substance we need for making cell membranes, for making steroid hormones, and for making bile. Cholesterol is carried in the bloodstream in packets known as lipoproteins and in recent years low density lipoproteins (LDL) have become known as carriers of saturated fats, animal fats. People most prone to atherosclerosis have excessive quantities of low density lipoproteins while people resistant to vascular disease have high concentrations of high density lipoproteins (HDL). What Brown and Goldstein found is that the cells of the body contain receptor mechanisms for taking up LDL and delivering it to the lysosomes (tiny cellular processing plants which use enzymes to break up the fatty particles into forms we can use for membranes and hormone manufacture). And when they identified the receptors for LDL, they learned that a high dietary intake of animal fats leads to the suppression of LDL receptors— apparently an overloading phenomenon—to such degree that excess LDL is left to circulate in the bloodstream, aggregating in areas where arterial injury has occurred, and forming a major part of an atheroma (also called an arterial plaque.)

This work earned a Nobel Prize in 1985 for Brown and Goldstein.

Some people seem to be genetically protected by possessing enough well-functioning LDL receptors to ensure they never build up large quantities of free-flowing cholesterol. Diet alterations can protect other people, for by limiting their intake of saturated and animal fats, they can attain the correct balance of LDL and LDL receptors for their particular bodies. Drugs are now available, as well, which block cholesterol synthesis. Some are lovastatin, compactin, mevinolin, and cholestyramine resin—the latter binding bile so that a portion of the cholesterol made in the liver is excreted and not recirculated.

In a now famous study, the Lipid Research Clinic followed 3806 healthy hypercholesterolemic men for an average of four to seven years, all of the men sticking to a low-cholesterol diet. A group of them, additionally, were treated with Questran, a cholestyramine resin, and the results were twenty-five percent less mortality from coronary heart disease, less angina, and less bypass surgery.

It is also believed that chronic injury caused to the blood vessels by the intense pressures of the blood flow results in a clotting mechanism playing a role in the formation of atheromas. When we break a blood vessel, whether the wound is through the skin or only under the skin, a blood clot forms. A clot on the inside of a vessel is technically called a thrombus. Like all clots, it is made of fibrin, a protein that helps flat platelet cells to cover the wound and stop the bleeding while the wound is healing. Platelets recognize a wound by sensing collagen that is exposed by the break in the vessel's endothelial lining. After the wound has healed, there is formation of scar tissue which dislodges the clot. Some of our white blood cells, called leukocytes, carry the clot away to be disposed of by enzymes. Enzymes dissolve the fibrin, thereby assisting in the breakup of the clot. We lose some of our quantity of such enzymes with age. Some clots then can fall away from a scar and, undissolved, flow freely through the blood until they lodge somewhere, blocking circulation. Such a clot is called an embolism; it is quite dangerous, often responsible for strokes and up to ninety percent of acute myocardial infarctions and sudden cardiac deaths are associated with occlusion of a coronary artery by a thrombus turned embolism.

Atherosclerotic plaques viewed through a microscope resemble an inflammatory reaction in some ways. They are like calluses which form on the skin as reactions to continual injury. Along with scar tissue, a plaque contains connective collagen and, often, lymphocytes. It then becomes a trap for phospholipids and polysaccharides—fats and sugars, and especially cholesterol—and thus it grows larger. Atheromas may result, then, from cumulative injuries to the blood vessels. And "injury" in this sense means not only an external blow to a blood vessel, but also the inevitable stress from the sheer pressure of blood flow—especially at junctions of the arteries. Blood pressure, it seems, causes constant injury in the arteries, begetting chronic inflammatory reactions, the forming of clots, which appear to lead to the formation of plaques. It is not unlike the way a river, swollen from heavy rains, erodes its banks, or the way a waterfall, over the years, eats into rock itself.

Occlusions and Dilations

Arterial blockages, which physicians call occlusions, occur most commonly in the aorta, the coronary arteries, the renal arteries, the common iliac or branching artery to the legs, the superficial femoral in the thigh, and in the carotid artery, better known as the jugular vein. The reasons for the occlusions may be atheromas, clots, a thrombus, an embolism, or a chronic spasm of an artery which makes it constrict, halting blood flow. An occluded coronary artery means that heart muscle dies, deprived of oxygen, and when such a condition is acute it is called myocardial infarction. If chronic, it is called ischemic heart disease. Angina pectoris is the chest pain felt when the heart does not receive enough oxygen to keep it going.

Treatment for blocked coronary arteries has expanded in recent years. Bypass surgery is simple in theory. You sew on a piece of artery in front and behind an occlusion, creating a detour for the blood. In practice, it is extremely delicate. Surgeons are well paid because they use great care and concentration on what they do. When you're handling someone's coronary arteries, your mind can't wander for a second. Pacemakers and implantable defibrillators compensate for heart beat irregularities by providing an electrical impulse to restore rhythm or even heart beat itself. A fibrillating heart has got its signals crossed, its signals, that is, to pump blood from the atrium to the ventricle or from the ventricle to the aorta.

Small balloons are sometimes used to unclog arteries when vasodilating drugs cannot do the job. They are inserted by catheter in an arm or in the groin and inflated when positioned just before the occlusion. In effect, the balloon expands the artery so the blood can pass over the clog.

It has been found that coronary artery occlusions are often caused not by lodged objects such as clots or atheromas, but by nervous system impulse errors or irregularities. Nerve impulses regulate constriction and dilation of the coronary arteries through "alpha" and "beta" receptors, respectively. Sometimes the signals go awry and the alphas predominate, closing off the arteries. Drugs called alpha blockers can prevent the constriction and beta blockers have the opposite effect—they prevent the artery from dilating. A third type of drugs, the calcium blockers, are beginning to be used to prevent spasms by controlling heart muscle contraction. If calcium cannot enter the muscle cells, the contractile proteins cannot touch each other to make the muscles work.

Aneurysms occur usually in the abdominal aorta in the area just before its branching into the iliac arteries. A balloon-like swelling, an aneurysm is a pouch of partially stalled blood causing the heart to pump harder to maintain total circulation. For many years, aneurysms were thought to be due to atherosclerosis, but now an inherited protein defect is believed the culprit, resulting in a failure of structural cross-linking in the affected vessel area. They may also, more simply, be due to years and years of the blood's pulsatile stress. Often, an aneurysm remains small and is never symptomatic, discovered only during autopsy. But when there is great swelling and danger of rupture, surgical nylon prosthesis is usually needed—a reinforcing jacket sewn around the artery.

There are hopeful signs on the heart's horizon which no doubt will mean cardiovascular disease mortality will continue to decline. Many scientists and physicians predict further breakthroughs in treatment and prevention, and drugs such as TPA that dissolve cloggage caused by clots are being improved. Longitudinal studies will soon yield fact, not theory, showing definitively how diet and exercise can intelligently be planned and pursued to prevent cardiovascular disease and, possibly, premature aging of the vessels. Exercise raises HDL serum levels and prolonged exercise appears to aid the body's clearing away of fatty deposits (as shown in an interesting Brown University study of long-distance runners reported in late 1986 in the Journal of the American Medical Association).

Transplanting healthy hearts for diseased ones was miraculous not very long ago. The main drawback was, and is, the body's rejection of material not made of its own tissue. The immune system, our great protector, knows what is "self" and what is "non-self." But geneticists are slowly unravelling the secrets of DNA's coil and they look forward to the day when we may analyze a person's cells to see his disease susceptibilities. Can the genetic code be redrawn to eliminate those susceptibilities? Yes, probably. The technical constraints of gene manipulation are not so formidable as the ethical problems which arise.

Chapter 10

Our Great Protector

The immune system is born with an ability to educate itself. It can recognize a danger, it can devise defense, and it can remember (when necessary) which defense to use for which danger.

However, this complex system of vigilant cells, our great protector from disease, changes after we reach maturity in ways that make us more susceptible to infectious disease.

More than one quarter of all people over 70 years old die of septicemia or pneumonia, infections which often go unnoticed, at least in the early stages. Elderly people, generally, have a somewhat lower normal body temperature, so a degree or two from a fever may not be detected.

Many specialized defenses are weakened in very elderly people, defenses such as coughing, ciliary action, and normal intestinal flora. Coughing not only is symptomatic of an infection; it aids in expelling invading antigens. Cilia, the waving, hairlike appendages on cells in the respiratory system, also aid in removing intruders, and intestinal bacteria defend the body by secreting substances that turn away other, unwanted, bacteria. These normally functioning defenses weaken in elderly people who have become immobile because of bad health or, many times, because of choice. Many drugs older people take can mask a fever, and diseases such as diabetes and cancer also impair the febrile response, as physicians call a fever. Another leading cause of death in people over 70 is cancer, and a reduction in immunologic

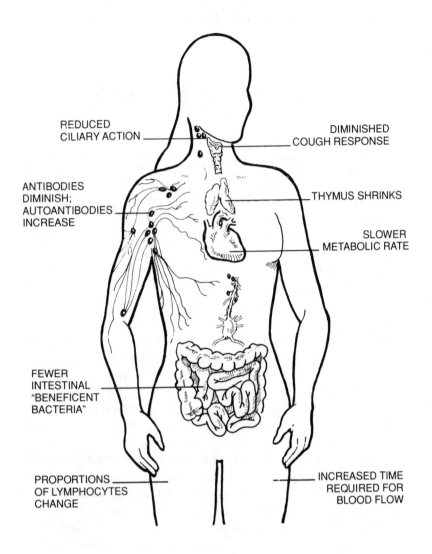

REDUCED
CILIARY ACTION

DIMINISHED
COUGH RESPONSE

ANTIBODIES
DIMINISH;
AUTOANTIBODIES
INCREASE

THYMUS SHRINKS

SLOWER
METABOLIC RATE

FEWER
INTESTINAL
"BENEFICENT
BACTERIA"

PROPORTIONS
OF LYMPHOCYTES
CHANGE

INCREASED TIME
REQUIRED FOR
BLOOD FLOW

Figure 18 The changing immune system

regulation means that cell growth that turns cancerous may go unchecked. Indeed, the body's immune defense fails to recognize simple antigens as skin test studies in people over 80 years old illustrate. Up to seventy percent of them react negatively to most skin tests. But, in addition to a decline in immunocompetence, the immune system may actually turn some of its components on us, attacking the body with autoimmune diseases like rheumatoid arthritis and multiple sclerosis.

Immune reduction brings to mind the theories of aging. Are these losses of immune regulation due to the wear and tear of a lifetime, the accumulation of genetic mutations which confuse the cells' functions? Is the immune system the seat of our biological clock, turning off its protection at a scheduled time? Or is it the evolutionary principle that guides the regulation of good health? Is protection summarily withdrawn from us once we are past our sexual maturity and child-rearing days since we have already done our part to continue the species? Since evolution (or more correctly, the species) no longer needs us, are we then cast out, so to speak, into the storm, braving the elements as best we can until, eventually, we succumb?

Man's particular evolutionary talent lies in his intelligence, the uses of his brain to overcome obstacles that are set up in his way. We like to improve things. We have devised adjustments for some aging changes in the form of corrective eye lenses, hearing aids, and implantable pacemakers. Through our social programs which help pay for medical care, we have made it possible for most people to take advantage of these adjustments. Many scientists believe that one of the greatest challenges for mankind today is to discover the detailed workings of the immune system. For learning how it protects us and when and why its functions wane, we will find ways through "immunoengineering" to restore and even prolong immunity and good health. Ways will be learned to overthrow the chronic, degenerative diseases that disable people for long periods of time in their late years. Some scientists commit ageism when they speak hopefully of techniques of "rejuvenating" the immune system, techniques such as bone marrow transplants, antiviral genetic engineering, and thymus hormone replacement. The ability to prolong immunity, wonderful as it will be, will not prevent us from aging. We will still have dry skin and gray hair. And we'll die some day. But when we learn to bolster the natural vaccines of our immune system, the catastrophic diseases of old age probably will go the way of smallpox and polio. Molecular biology has already begun to produce medical techniques for enhancing immunity, for fighting infections and cancer, and for suppressing autoimmunity in the fight against diseases such as arthritis. Scientists have begun to manufacture the hybridoma, a cross between a cancerous cell and a strong anti-cancer immune cell, and they are hopeful of bolstering the immune system with such so-called "monoclonal antibodies."

The development of the smallpox vaccine in the late eighteenth century came after natural immunity was discovered. Edward Jenner theorized that the reason milkmaids did not contract smallpox was because they had been sick with a similar but less harmful disease, cowpox. He injected fluid from a milkmaid's cowpox sore into a child and, sometime later, injected the same child with fluid from a smallpox sore. The child proved to be immune to smallpox. His immune system had learned a defense against the disease because of his inoculation with similar antigens. Our researchers now have a clearer, if incomplete, picture of our remarkable immune system. They create vaccines from microorganisms that have been altered to produce an immune response but not full blown disease. These "attenuated" microbes cannot multiply, perhaps, or they have been weakened from growing many cycles in laboratory culture. They are another example of man-made adjustments like hearing aids and false teeth, allowing us to age in good health.

Regulation of Immunity

What specifically occurs in the regulatory role of the immune system as it ages with the rest of the body? What are the changes in this declining watch dog of our health, resulting in less natural protection for us as we grow older? Why do we grow more susceptible to viral and bacterial disease, to the growth of tumors, and to autoimmunity? There are four ways immune deficiency can happen: It may be inherited, it may be acquired through illness, it may be iatrogenic (temporary deficiency stemming from drug thereapy), or it may come simply from growing old. It is helpful to consider first the changes that occur in the aging immune system, for that sets the stage for a basic understanding of its mechanisms, most of which may be seen only by microscopic multi-magnification.

The loss of proper regulation is the most significant of all the changes of our aging bodies, and in the immune system, regulation is the key word. Changes in metabolism, in blood flow, in the size of our organs, in the proportions of lean mass to fat mass, in the strength of our bones, and in the nervous and endocrine systems all challenge the regulatory capacity of the immune system. It must adjust its protective functions to keep in step with the changing requirements of home-ostasis. But it must do its job with less of its own resources, for it, too, loses "mass." The loss is chiefly in the size of the thymus, a glandlike organ at the base of the neck, just behind the top of the sternum, sitting, as it were, on the top of the heart. The role of the thymus in immunity is rather like a school—some of the white blood cells called lymphocytes spend time there gaining the knowledge for fighting specific diseases. The thymus begins to shrink about the time of our sexual maturity. Its cortex, about eighty percent of its mass when we are children, involutes rapidly and accounts for only about twenty-four percent of the thymus by the time we are 35 or 40. Secretions of thymic hormones, thymosin in particular, which help to stimulate an immune response, diminish along with the size of the thymus. Some scientists argue that by the time we are capable of reproduction, we have been exposed to most disease antigens and so there is no longer a need for the education of the immune system's cells. But some scientists do not believe this and they point out other changes in the system, detrimental to immunity, which seem to be related to the changing role of the thymus.

Lymphocytes, once they have learned how to recognize disease, wait for battle, like soldiers in their barracks, in many places of the body. The spleen is one such barracks and it loses relatively little of its size over the years. The lymph nodes also are storage sites and there are many of these, including the tonsils and the adenoids, located near the body's orifices where infection commonly enters. The abdomen is full of lymph nodes. Lymph nodes swell when we have an infection, because the troops of lymphocytes are multiplying into battalions, making ready to confront the invading threat. During aging, neither the nodes nor the numbers of lymphocytes decrease very much, although the types of lymphocytes do change. Old people have fewer "killer" cells and they have more "suppressor" cells than "helper" cells. These cells form what is known as the cellular arm of immunity. Since it is in the thymus that the cells of immunity learn their specific roles as killers, helpers, or suppressors, the loss of regulation in their proportions seems likely due to the reduced mass of the thymus.

The proteins called antibodies or immunoglobulins (another very important component of the immune system) circulate in the bloodstream. Their role is to provide our other arm of the immune response—the humoral or fluid arm, ridding most infectious agents from our bodies before we even know we have been invaded. They also have a connection to the thymus and their numbers decline slightly as we age. This means we are less well-buttressed against infectious diseases and explains why pneumonia and viral influenzas plague older people and can be so deadly. When the immune system is in good order, it meets infection by what is called amplification—a boost of its defensive forces. But the opposite of amplification is suppression. When regulation is out of kilter, for reasons our scientists do not yet understand, the immune system suppresses its forces. This allows infections to go unchallenged.

As numbers of antibodies diminish, their opposite, auto-antibodies, may increase in number. Fighters which mistake our own body parts for antigen agents which do not belong, autoantibodies are the culprits of autoimmunity and their appearance in the blood is, again, the result of a loss of proper regulation.

Autoimmunity is a result of extreme amplification of the system. Mistaking cells of the body as agents of disease, the system amplifies its production of autoantibodies. In rheumatoid arthritis, these autoantibodies attack and destroy the integrity of the bone joints, commonly in the hands, feet, legs, and the jaw. The accompanying swelling (called inflammation) is due to dilation of the blood vessels by large migrations of white blood cells and antibodies to the affected areas. Multiple sclerosis is another disease believed to be associated with autoimmunity. Actually, its origin is thought to be a slow acting virus that changes its "host" cell into a different form, attracting autoantibodies. They destroy the myelin insulation of nerve cells, forming scars or plaques in the brain. The disorder is more common in women than men, and is an age-onset disease rather than a disease of old age. Usually it begins before the age of 40.

Autoimmunity is also a factor of lupus erythematosus which affects people (usually women) younger than 35. Its cause is thought to be a lack of recognition by some immune cells for others, a loss of regulation that results in an attack on cellular DNA, among other cellular structures. Atherosclerosis, the disease of the blood vessels, has a component of white blood cell infiltration. Lymphocytes congregate on the atheromas, the fat deposits, perhaps assisting in the formation of plaques.

Cancer can develop and spread when the immune system's regulation favors its own suppression. A cancerous cell is one whose proper structure has been altered. Perhaps a genetic mutation causes it, or it has changed its form, as in multiple sclerosis, due to a slowly acting virus. We probably form cancerous cells throughout our lives, but the immune system, through its monitoring function called immune surveillance, seems to recognize cancerous cells as abnormal and then destroys them. Cancer occurs with its highest frequency in children and in old people. So it is theorized that, in children with leukemia, immune surveillance is not yet completely developed and in older people it has lost its regulatory powers. Another theory has it that cancer is the result of an accumulation of cell mutations—perhaps from external irritants like fumes, radiation, and pesticides, or from slow viruses which transform the cells they inhabit. But since such carcinogens do not commonly result in cancer in young adults, it seems logical to conclude that an age-related decline in immune regulation is the reason the disease develops so often in older adults.

Education of the Cells

When you take a few ounces of blood and spin the fluid for a few minutes in a laboratory centrifuge, you will separate it into two layers of cells, the dense red blood cells resting under a ring of white blood cells. Actually, the cells on top are not white, but clear when you look at them through a microscope. They are some of the immune system's lymphocytes and they are quite well educated—for cells. They have the basic knowledge of all cells such as how to divide and where to go within that universe of a human body to perform their particular reason for being. But they know a lot more. As they patrol the interior of the body, they touch other cells and they know whether a cell is "self" (that is, part of the body) or "non-self" (a particle that does not belong because it is not a part of the body).

When the immune system finds non-self matter (an act called antigen-recognition) it unleashes some extraordinary powers, particularly the lymphocytes. Depending on the specific type of lymphocyte it is (and there are many types) it may gobble up the invader in a single, surrounding engulfment, it may fire off a chemical poison to neutralize the enemy, it may trigger its own doubling, many times over, and it may release an enzymatic alarm, calling its lymphocytic brothers-in-arms to hurry to the scene of battle.

All our cells learn differentiation. They learn early whether they are heart cells, intestinal cells, brain cells, spleen cells, skin cells, or blood vessel cells. They learn their functions when we are just embryos and then fetuses. As the parts and organs form, however, there is not yet an immune reaction—our mother's immune protection extends to us—but after organogenesis and growth, when we are more or less ready for birth, our immune system starts to come into its own. It knows the characteristics of all our other systems and it knows right from wrong. As our great protector, its job is to recognize whatever does not belong and then get rid of it. Without a knowledgeable immune system, we could not face the host of pollen, viral, bacterial, and parasitic challenges our world presents.

The reason that organ transplants meet so little success is that the immune system rejects them as non-self matter. The new organ does not have the same genetic and molecular characteristics of its new host unless it is from an identical twin, and the immune system, though it can be suppressed by drugs for a time, will usually reject the non-self tissue. The development of synthetic material that is used in pacemakers and hip joints came only after laborious research to find inert material that does not provoke an immune reaction.

We learn to live with many bacteria and, in fact, make use of them. In our mouth, bacteria help our enzymes begin to break down foods into nutrients and others do similar services for us in our stomach and intestine. Our immune system provides a low-grade reaction to these types of bacteria but it has even learned to hold back its full-scale, inflammatory defense, since besides aiding our digestion, some of the bacteria take on immune support roles themselves. They fight off many pathogens for us. The immune system winks at them, almost considering them "self" but not quite, because it never lets them get inside the body. They must stay on the surface of the skin, the mouth, or the intestine. If they should attempt to move through the epithelial cell layer, the immune system will sound the alarm and go after them.

A Digression Into Molecular Warfare

An immune reaction is an orchestrated defense with specific events: recognition of the invader, learning how to overpower it, and the actual battle. When a flu virus enters the body, it commandeers a cell, substituting its DNA code for our own. It replicates, using our RNA apparatus, and then tries to take over as many cells as it can. The immune system first combats the flu with macrophages, white blood cells that try to eat anything that is non-self. Macrophages also signal for cells called granulocytes to gather nearby and release histamine. Histamine is a chemical signal for openings to form in the blood vessel walls, setting free a flood of lymphocytes and other white blood cells. This influx of fluid causes the swelling, edema, in the area of infection.

So far, the reaction is a first line defense. The release of histamines in the nasal cavities is what causes us to sneeze. Allergies are usually reactions like this. The immune system attacks an invading agent, such as pollen, as if it were a virus and sometimes an allergic reaction includes a host of lymphocytes that cause swelling or rashes.

Usually, an invader gets no farther than this initial reaction. We sneeze a time or two and that's that. But sometimes a virus is a strong one, or one we have not fought before, and our initial defense must be supplemented. This is the time for education of the lymphocytes: A macrophage takes a virus it has engulfed to the thymus where in a classroom environment they learn the invader's characteristics by feeling it. This process, antigen recognition, is only part one of the lesson; after they have learned about the enemy which they are going to fight, the lymphocytes are then given assignments and are taught specific roles. Some of them become "B cells" and they circulate in the bloodstream secreting antibodies. Others become "T cells" and differentiate even further as killers, helpers, and suppressors. The two types of cells then leave the thymus and create a two-armed immune response; the B cell response of antibodies in the bloodstream is our humoral immunity and the T cell response is our cellular immunity. With aging comes a reduction in the proportions of these cells, so we usually have fewer killer and helper cells, but more suppressors. And most important is the fact that it takes longer for the system to respond in an old person who is in trouble when infection progresses faster than the immune system can respond.

Antibodies can cover a virus, neutralizing it so it can no longer penetrate or infect cells. Humoral immunity includes the helper T cells which assist the antibodies by providing a stimulus for their production. The antibodies do not actually kill the virus, but they cover its receptor mechanism so it cannot enter a cell. Then, through a chemical process called complement activity, the antibody attracts enzymes similar to digestive enzymes which arrive and dissolve the virus.

Killer T cells speed from the thymus to the lymph nodes and the spleen where they rapidly proliferate. The job of the killer T cells is to destroy the cells already infected by the virus—a very important and crucial task, for it strikes the disease at its source. Lymph nodes bulge with lymphocytes during infections, many for the attack, many to make antibodies, and many as reserves or memory cells. Physicians stopped removing swollen tonsils routinely a few decades ago, as scientists discovered their importance as storage sites of the lymph system.

The battle won, there are different types of cells which provide clean-up. They remove the debris of cells that lysed from the viral invasion, and some of them form scar tissue to protect the sites of injury while new tissue forms. Some of the victorious B and T cells return to the lymph nodes where they wait for the next time the same flu will invade. They will keep their memory of the virus for as long as twenty-five or thirty years, sometimes longer. Recognition, education, and memory are not only functions of our brain, but also of our immune system's cells.

Bone marrow is quite an important part of the immune system, the birthplace of the cells of immunity. All of our blood cells, both red and white, come from stem cells in the calcified, internal centers of the bones, strong, well protected areas. Even when bones decalcify with old age, the stem cells continue to divide, producing as many white cells for us as ever (although when the disease chips are down, they do not function as well). A great mystery in biology is what, exactly, tells a spherical stem cell, deep within a bone, to divide and become a white blood cell, or a red blood cell, or an osteocyte, a bone cell. Victims of anemia have some inborn error in this bone marrow cell metabolism. They either do not produce enough red blood cells, or the ones they make are defective, fated to lyse soon after dividing.

Vaccinations against infectious diseases commonly use dead or otherwise altered viral matter and the immune system thus gets its education by examining harmless antigens. This is called the primary reaction. A secondary reaction, which takes a much shorter period of time, occurs when B and T cells rapidly divide and go out after the invader when it infects the body the second time. Why do we get the flu so often? Why does the immune system fail to remember it and combat it as soon as we have been re-infected? Well, we rarely get the same flu virus twice. The pesky organism

1. FIRST LINE DEFENSE

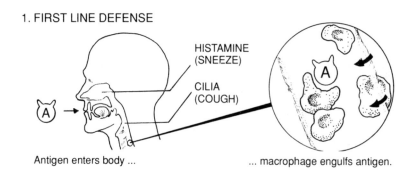

HISTAMINE
(SNEEZE)

CILIA
(COUGH)

Antigen enters body ...   ... macrophage engulfs antigen.

2. EDUCATION AND MEMORY

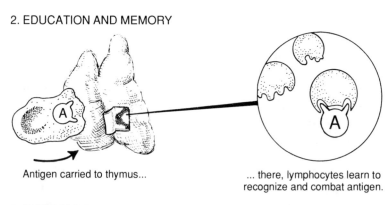

Antigen carried to thymus...   ... there, lymphocytes learn to
                                          recognize and combat antigen.

3. THE BATTLE

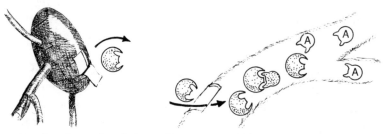

Lymph nodes produce "educated"   ... which then circulate and destroy
lymphocytes ...   antigen invaders. Afterward, some of
                                         the victorious lymphocytes return to
                                         the nodes and stand ready, for
                                         years, to meet the enemy again.

Figure 19 The immune reaction

mutates every few years or so and it invades us in a changed form, one the immune system must learn to combat all over again. Many so-called "staph" infections have evolved a defense allowing them to hide from the white blood cells. These staphylococcus bacteria contain a protein that lets them actually attach to antibodies. The antibodies cover them, but without incapacitating them, and so lymphocytes and other antibodies do not know they are there. This is the sort of infection requiring an antibiotic drug, a chemical killer that works independently of the immune system.

Why do herpes viruses stay with us so long? This is a rather undemanding predator, content to sit quiescent in an epithelial cell for long periods. Occasionally, something will activate it, perhaps the sunlight hits it or we touch the spot, or we fall into a period of stress or depression, and the virus starts growing. Then the immune system goes after it and eventually the infectious process is under control once again.

One theory for the aging increase in our number of autoantibodies (the culprits of multiple sclerosis and rheumatoid arthritis) is related to the herpes type of virus. Some scientists believe that viruses may begin to transform their host cells after a long dormant time. The immune system makes antibodies to attack these transformed cells, recognized as non-self, and in the process, they attack healthy cells which resemble the diseased ones. So the "slow virus" may be causing us many of our old age diseases in addition to cancer.

Besides the new herpes fighting drug, acyclovir, it appears that we soon will have a vaccine for some forms of herpes. Recombinant-DNA technology allows scientists to create an artificial virus with characteristics of the real thing, but without the virulent properties. Such a product, when injected and studied by the immune system so that we will have the ability to defend ourselves with secondary reactions, is another of the reasons genetic engineering is going to help us as we age.

Immunogenetics

The immune system, still obscure just a few years ago, has fast become a household phrase. Researchers are unravelling its secrets surely, and not too slowly, now that they have gained a grip on genetics in general. The immune system is more difficult to observe than the palpable muscular or cardiovascular systems. It has parts, to be sure, that are easily seen—its "organs" such as the thymus, spleen, and lymph nodes—but our growing knowledge of its molecular and cellular components and activities is due to our ability, now, to examine it from the viewpoint of molecular biology, a viewpoint that has become possible since DNA was described. Gigantic textbooks now present immune system details that were totally unknown five years ago. Still, there is far more that is not known.

Immunodeficiency is a term that has moved from medical texts to newspapers and television, primarily in news stories about medical attempts to improve the lives of children who are sadly born with immunodeficiency or with adults, the victims of AIDS, who have an acquired immune deficiency syndrome. Finding a vaccine or a cure for AIDS is a woefully difficult task and, in the early 1980s at least, a woefully neglected one by those who held the research purse-strings. The virus causing AIDS changes form, in the manner of flu viruses, so creating a vaccine that can stimulate antibody response to all its forms is a formidable challenge. There can be no doubt that ways to reverse AIDS and other immune deficiency diseases will be found. It is a question of priorities. Experimental therapy became big news in late 1986 when some AIDS victims seemed to benefit from a drug called AZT (currently known as Retrovir) which, if not a cure, apparently slowed the disease process. Concentrated efforts are underway in several countries for not only developing an AIDS vaccine, but also for testing it on people. At the same time, many scientists are reordering research priorities, realizing that huge outlays of society's funds in "wars" on cancer or other specific diseases are like trying to put the roof on a building before laying the foundation. Foremost among those asking for basic, rather than specialized research, is Lewis Thomas, chancellor of Memorial Sloan-Kettering Cancer Center, who notes that most of the great advances in science were discovered as almost accidental by-products of basic research.

The word coming from basic immunology research is hopeful. Ways of delaying the immune system's loss of regulation, of restoring its declining function, and of correcting immunodeficiencies are seen as probabilities rather than as dreams. Geneticists are zeroing in on a segment of DNA, chromosome six, where they have identified a group of genes called the major histocompatibility complex (MHC). Evidence has mounted that the immune response to antigens, or disease susceptibility itself, is controlled there. If you're going to manipulate genes, MHC is the group of genes you want to learn about.

Genetics has made it possible to discover the oncogene, an important key to understanding cancer. J. Michael Bishop has written in *Scientific American*, "What has been learned from oncogenes represents the first peep behind the curtain that for so long has obscured the mechanisms of cancer." An oncogene is a gene directing the construction of a protein that can alter the structure of a cell, thus it contains the potential to cause cancer and it appears that point mutations caused by molecular matter such as radiation or chemicals, or the virus family known as retroviruses, may activate this potential. Scientists have discovered more: Only a small number of cells in a malignant tumor actually metastasize and these few cells contain specific proteins which seem to dictate whether metastasis will occur.

But genetics is not the only way to affect the immune system. Manipulating diet is easier. And many experiments with mice have zeroed in on fats and protein as perpetrators of autoimmunity. Robert A. Good of the University of Oklahoma is one scientist who has reported an enhanced immune response in mice on diets with restrictions on fats and proteins. Mice given a diet heavy with fats and protein came down with diseases earlier than those fed normally. Dr. Good has also found that a zinc deficiency is related to the loss of immune regulation—the mineral seems to support T cell immunity. He says, "We may begin to look forward to a time when dietary manipulation may be incorporated into treatment or even prevention of the diseases of aging."

Evidence illustrating how depression and stress harm the immune system—therefore making us easier prey to disease—has been appearing lately in medical journals. A study, for example, at Mt. Sinai School of Medicine in New York showed that lymphocytes are suppressed in clinical depression. Following a group of men whose wives had died, researchers found that the men's ability to respond to infections declined significantly during their bereavement, and their weakened immunity persisted as long as a year. Other researchers have found that university students' helper T cells and killer T cells are reduced in numbers during the stress of studying for final exams. And, of course, stress stimulates secretions of adrenalcorticotrophic hormone which, in turn, stimulates steroid hormones whose effects include immune suppression.

In fact, the effects of drugs and hormones on the immune system are being studied by many researchers. Immunosuppressive drugs are used in skin grafts and organ transplant operations, not always successfully, to be sure, and they leave patients easy prey to infection while keeping the immune system's power to reject the transplant at bay. But some scientists, such as Takashi Makinodan of the Geriatric Research, Educational and Clinical Center of the Veterans Administration, are hopeful that drugs which will destroy autoantibodies and leave other immune functions intact will soon be commonly used. Thymic hormones are being studied as potential stimulators of stem cells to form T and B fighter cells.

Surgical methods to bolster immunity are more in the planning stage now than the stage of success. But they, too, hold a potential and are being explored: bone marrow transplants or the actual injection of young bone marrow cells and thymus gland tissue into old bodies; removal of the thymus or spleen if they prove to be the source of autoantibodies or viral-induced cancer growth; and the freezing and preservation of lymphocytes, when we are young, for injection when we are old.

More at hand for us now is a far less complicated way to keep the immune system in good order. Exercise can help, as it helps all our bodily systems. The cells of the immune system need strong bones for their protection and growth, and an unimpeded blood flow to help them when they must travel to the sites of infection. Good blood flow, which regular exercise builds, helps us in another way, also important for the immune system. It makes it easier to rid the body of "immune complexes"—antibodies which have engulfed antigens—so they, as debris, do not clog the kidneys. It is no coincidence that sedentary people often develop kidney disease. Flushing the immune system of its debris is another reason why drinking plenty of water is helpful.

Many scientists believe that the site of the biological clock in the body, a clock that ticks away the years in a planned schedule, lies in the thymus. When the thymus loses its size, they point out, we become progressively weaker against disease until one day, a particular disease overpowers us.

As it happens, the thymus is not calling the shots. The thymus gets its instructions from a higher source, the brain, the body's control center. That is where we should look for a biological clock.

Chapter 11

The Body's Control Center

For most people aging brings anxiety. We expend precious energy fretting over worrisome questions. Will we lose our physical strength and spend our old age chronically battling bad health? Will we lead boring, isolated years outside society, cut off from the concerns where our energy was better expended—family, career colleagues, friends? Will we become remorseful and depressed, wishing we had followed different paths in life, embittered at the adjustments our changed position makes necessary? Perhaps the most frightening worry of all is that we might lose our intellect. Will aging mean diminishing mental ability, the loss of memory, sleepless nights, days or years of dependency on uncaring nurses in the bewildering environment of the old folks' home?

These questions should not give us fear, for the answer to them is no. They are attitudes of ageism, not facts of biological aging. Mental impairment is not an inevitable change of age; depression, boredom and loneliness need not be ways of adjusting to a changed position.

The human brain and our central nervous system, said to contain as many as two hundred trillion cells, control not only our intellect, of course. The brain coordinates nearly everything about us from our autonomic nervous system which masterminds our involuntary movements—breathing, digestion, reflexes, hormonal regulation, immune defense—

to our rational power to assess and decide our personal responses to life's challenges. Aging is accompanied by adjustments in our hormone levels, major movers in the body's regulation, and most of these changes are coordinated by releasing factors from the brain, signals from the hypothalamus giving the pituitary gland instructions to change the hormonal balance. The brain is a control center *par excellence*. It knows when homeostatic mechanisms need adjustments because the body's nerve cells and hormones, the neuroendocrine teamwork, constantly supply status reports. Whether the brain or the endocrine glands are causal in hormonal pathogenesis is rather like the old question, which comes first, the chicken or the egg?

The brain's controlling job is immense, almost as unfathomable to our understanding as two hundred trillion nerve cells, called neurons. What an organizer the brain is. Inevitably, we lose some neurons as we age but the loss occurs only in some parts of the brain and not in others. When we damage nerve cells, their long axons can regenerate. And they grow back quickly, about as fast as a healthy fern frond.

But senility is neither inevitable nor untreatable. Our culture has until now equated old age with senility, a form of age prejudice assuming that old people are forgetful, slow-thinking, confused, and, more often than not, cranky in temper.

Western society has assumed also more often than not, that old age is a sad time for people, a burdensome time for their families. Recently, some pessimists have begun to call our increasing numbers of elderly people an economic burden for the tax-paying public. It is no wonder that people grow old believing that age in itself is depressing. What is truly sad is that when many of them become depressed, it is likely due to a physical ailment which could be treated if physicians were not so ready to assume "old age senility" and look no further in their diagnosis. Much confusion has been caused in old people by modern medicine—drugs—a fact that physicians and family members only recently have begun to realize.

The good news in brain research is that senility does not have to be a part of the aging process. We can change our attitudes now that science is explaining the biochemical changes in the central nervous system. Nowadays and in the future, when we forget where we parked our car our physicians will likely relate our confusion to a physical problem, arteriosclerosis, say, rather than senility, and treat it so that blood flow is restored to the part of the brain controlling memory. We are learning that the brain functions very well for most people who reach ripe old age; the true organic disorders like senile dementia, Alzheimer's disease, and Parkinson's disease are in reality infrequent occurrences. Less than five percent of people over 65 ever have senile dementia in any form and most of them suffer mildly or moderately. Even better news is that our growing knowledge of how the brain communicates and ages with the body is giving us ways to treat these dreaded neurological diseases—with very hopeful success rates.

Brain research is an idea whose time is overdue. Soon, the census takers tell us, one of every five Americans will be over 65. Even now, people in their seventies and eighties may be the fastest-growing proportion of the population. More additions to life expectancy and better health for old people are the results of research. But research doesn't get done for free. Besides allocating a larger part of society's resources to continuing and improving this research, we can do more to assure mental and neurological health in our individual old age. Because the brain and nervous system are physical parts of the body like the rest of our systems, their health depends on exercise and proper diet. Vigorous physical exercise promotes good blood circulation, keeping oxygen flowing to the brain, and, also important, clearing waste away before it can create harm such as tangling some vital neurons. Physical exercise is no less vital for the brain than it is for keeping the kidneys clear. Common sense tells us that mental exercise also keeps the brain healthy. Science is confirming it.

Matters of White and of Gray

Another which comes first, the chicken or the egg? question rises in considering blood flow to the brain in old people. If blood flow is reduced or obstructed, brain cells starve and die just as all oxygen-deprived cells anywhere in the body. Atherosclerosis and blood clots can block the vessels supplying blood to the brain, causing cells to die, sometimes damaging brain tissue to such an extent (as in a stroke) that the victim may lose some movement, sensory or speech functions, or may develop senile dementia symptoms. Most people in Western society, as many as ninety percent of people over 75 years old, have atherosclerosis to some degree. And arterial stiffening, with adjustments in blood pressure, is a universal and progressive change of our aging bodies. So reduced blood flow to the brain can be said to be an aging change, although it is a change not originating in the brain itself. It is a change in the cardiovascular system that affects the brain.

For the same reasons that the last two decades have witnessed a decline in mortality from heart disease, that is, less cigarette smoking, more exercise, and more attention to diet, the incidence of stroke, too, has declined in the United States.

From the early Fifties to the late Seventies, cerebrovascular accident caused by arterial blockages, dislodged blood clots, or hemorrhage has struck fewer people. Statistics vary widely, but some reports claim that the stroke rate has dropped almost fifty percent.

Even in the absence of arteriosclerosis and cardiovascular disease, blood flow to the brain is reduced in old people. Why? The brain regulates blood flow to itself as it regulates the flow to the other organs, and it is not greedy; it only takes what it needs. The aging brain gets smaller, not alarmingly so, but by about ten percent by age 80, and therefore all its chemical metabolism is reduced by about the same percentage. So the brain itself makes an adjustment in its own blood supply, since it no longer needs as much as it once did.

The brain's shrinkage is thought to be the result of a lifetime's loss of neurons, the nerve cells. Cell loss is a normal, indeed, a fundamental change of aging in the human body, most organs losing some size by the time we are 70 or 80. Like the other organs, the brain has a large reserve capacity, able to continue functioning just fine even when it loses ten or twelve percent of its weight. Although we do not yet know why, "gray matter," several layers of neurons which form a mantle around the brain, undergoes a faster rate of cell loss between the ages of 20 and 50 than does the "white matter," the inner mass of the brain. After age 50, however, the loss rates change proportion, the white matter shrinking more than the gray. The cerebrum, cerebellum, and spinal cord all share in the shrinking process, but there is no evidence yet that the hypothalamus, the control center for hormonal regulation, changes size.

White matter and gray matter are so named because of a difference in the myelin surrounding nerve cells. A neuron has a bulky body, called the nerve cell body, with its own nucleus, DNA, and protein production sites. The nerve cell's long axon, the part we call a nerve, is surrounded by an insulation or membrane of lipid or fat cells, called glial cells or myelin. The more myelin surrounding a nerve cell, the whiter its appearance, and the interior of the brain is white because it is well-insulated. A reason we need fatty acids and other cholesterol-producing nutrients in our diet is because they are essential materials for the synthesis of cell membranes in general and nerve cell insulation in particular. If myelin is not made in sufficient quantity or if it is destroyed, for example, by too much alcohol, the signals that are being transmitted through the nerve cells can misfire or short-circuit, leading to uncontrolled, tremor-like movements or, worse, irrational thinking.

The fact that we all lose neurons adds substance to the

genetic theory of aging. Our loss of neurons is certainly not random. It appears that some parts of the brain lose no neurons, or very few, during aging, while other parts lose many, as many in fact, as fifty percent. Thus neuronal loss is selective and those who believe in the biological clock theory can point to this as evidence that certain nervous system functions are programmed to wane. Recent technological improvements in looking at the brain, computerized axial tomography scanning and nuclear magnetic resonance, have allowed scientists to discover the selectiveness of neuronal loss. They have seen, for instance, that certain areas of the brain, chiefly those concerned with posture and movement, maintain the same number of cells throughout a long life. The areas of greatest cell loss seem to be the frontal and temporal regions, and one spot, the *locus ceruleus,* which is thought to have some control over our sleep patterns.

Aging indisputably brings changes in our sleep patterns. We wake up during the night and blame it on tension, but perhaps the irregularity is related to the loss of neurons. Researchers have found that the time spent in deep sleep and REM sleep (which means rapid-eye-movement) decreases as we age. A lack of deep sleep has obvious implications for our mental health as well as our personal disposition. If some old people become grouchy, maybe it is because they cannot get enough sleep. Many old people find they need naps during the day—aging seems to indicate more sleep is needed than when we are young—because they wake up during the night and are unable to return to sleep. Evidently, some nursing home staffers have not been apprised of current research, for it is reported that they do not allow their patients to nap in the afternoon. The reason they do not allow daytime sleeping is because they believe it is responsible for the patients' inability to sleep at night, an inconvenience to staffers who would rather watch late night television movies than tend to patients' needs.

Estimates of neuronal loss in the visual cortex portion of the brain range to fifty percent and many old people need eyesight adjustments. As we age, we need more light to see well and there are changes at work other than those in the brain. The human eye lens hardens, losing flexibility, and the general loss of muscular strength and coordination extends to the muscles of the eye. Cross-linking of the fibers in the lens increases, as it does in all connective tissue. In the extreme, this is the cause of opaqueness in the lens which may develop into a cataract. The condition is no longer a serious cause of blindness since improved removal techniques are successful most of the time.

Cell loss, a phenomenon of all aging in the body, does not exclude the eye structure, and reductions in blood supply affect our vision. Presbyopia or far-sightedness is a universal aging change, necessitating reading glasses for most people by the mid 40s. Increasing viscosity of the lens fluid takes responsibility, making it more difficult for the lens to change shape on focussing at a short distance. As we age, we also lose a slight bit of our field vision, the right and left-sided view we take in when looking straight ahead. Glaucoma, a result of intraocular pressure and a hardening lens, no longer is a serious threat to our sight as we grow old since it can be treated.

Other sensory losses of old people may be related to neuronal loss, although this is not proven. The loss of auditory function, particularly in the high frequency range, and the loss of our sense of balance, controlled in the inner ear, are also believed to be related to reduced blood flow—again, an arteriosclerosis connection. Almost one-third of all people who reach old age have a hearing difficulty and about one-tenth gain "biological noise"—tinnitus, periodic or sometimes constant ringing in the ears. A hearing aid amplifies sounds and voices for most hearing loss, and it can often ease the frustration of tinnitus. Some hearing loss can be prevented, such as neuronal loss from the acoustic trauma of occupational loud noise and recreational loud music.

Olfactory senses are usually reduced in old people, due mostly to a loss of smell and taste receptors in the nose and on the tongue. But this may also be related to a loss of neurons in the brain whose function it is to tell us what the smell and taste buds are reporting.

Neurotransmitters

Ever since we human beings realized that we differed from animals because of our ability to think, we have wanted to know how our brain works. It is the most intricate of all creations on earth, the most difficult to study and to explain. Following different paths and using dissimilar techniques, poets and scientists share the same dream of revealing the workings of the mind. Neither poet nor scientist, though, will piece the puzzle together on his own. The scientist will have soon described all the brain's components and he may even discover how to keep them all healthy and in good physical condition. He will never be able to explain why one person thinks one way while another thinks differently. That is the poet's realm. As many scientists admit, there is more to the human brain than biology.

These days some people speculate that man can devise a computer with the complex capabilities of the human brain. These people are neither scientists nor poets. They are business people and their goals are usually pursued more for profit potential than for answering philosophical longings. Making a mechanical brain is neither a poetic task nor, in scientific terms, a realistic objective. Even if we could produce a system of billions upon billions of human thought responses, how could we pack it all into several neat little cubic centimeters, the volume of our brain? There are limits to the size of silicon chips but if there are limits to the brain's capacity we are not aware of them.

Physical movements are the results of signals from the brain, stimulations of muscles by nerves. When muscles receive a stimulus, they allow calcium to enter to regulate contraction and extension. But what about the signal that originates in the brain? It is the result of thought. We feel an itch on our leg (because a nerve signal moves from leg to brain) and we have a thought: Scratch it. Admittedly less than profound, this thought translates into muscular movement, an accomplishment of biology just as profound in its way as man-devised philosophies, religions, and artistic achievements. How does the brain do this? The answer is that all those billions upon billions of neurons in the brain can communicate with each other electrochemically. And, it is believed, our thoughts themselves are results of a series of neurons stimulating each other until the information we have stored (memory) is associated with the new information we are putting in (cognition). All our thoughts are the results of cognition, memory, and association. We learn something, we store the knowledge, and we can retrieve the knowledge when we make an association with it. For example, when we eat an apple, we form a memory of color, shape, texture, taste. To the memory we add learned knowledge of nutritional value. Then when we see or bite into another apple, there sparks across our brain a series of electrochemical impulses through circuits of neurons, resulting in our association of what we see with our stored knowledge that it is something to be eaten.

The impulses shooting along through the nerves or through the brain's neurons, like electricity, owe their movement to a flow of sodium and potassium ions. Just as we need calcium for our muscles and a little fat to insulate our nerves, we need salt for the nerves to function. Other indispensable factors in neuronal communication are the neurotransmitters, molecules of hormones which carry the impulse from one neuron to the next. Our nerves are not continuous lengths of cell tissue, but are broken by synapses between each nerve cell so that no two nerves actually touch each other. Electrochemical impulses travel through the axon of a nerve and they halt at each nerve cell ending. For the impulse to cross to the next nerve cell it needs a bridge over the space called a synapse and Mother Nature designed the neurotransmitter to do this job in one of her usual strokes of economy. The neurotransmitters enable the impulses to go from one cell to another. As one scientist, Jan Klein, has put it, neurotransmitters are like "ferryboats carrying passengers across the river."

Neurotransmitters are made in the nerve cell body, packaged in little sacs called vesicles, and then they take up temporary residence at the nerve cell endings where there are many branches called dendrites. Here the neurotransmitters wait for an impulse. When it arrives, the sacs attach to the nerve cell membrane and pour out their neurotransmitter contents which diffuse across the synapse and bind to receptors on the neighboring nerve cell. They deliver the impulse, in short, which then continues on its way along another nerve cell. Meanwhile, the empty sacs travel back to their own nerve cell body and receive fresh neurotransmitters for their next mission.

Neurotransmitters are vital to our well-being. As messengers between the nerve cells, it is up to them whether the brain can communicate with the rest of the body. Without them, we would have no muscular movement—voluntary or involuntary. Besides our being immobilized, our lungs could not breathe and our heart could not beat. Neurotransmitters are pivotal in the endocrine system, for without them the brain's signals for hormonal releases would not be delivered. A fertilized egg would not last long in the ovary if the signal to shut down the menstrual cycle was stopped at the first nerve cell ending outside the hypothalamus. Without neurotransmitters we would not be able to see, to comprehend, to hear, or to think—but then, we would be dead.

Aging brings a reduction of some neurotransmitters in some parts of the brain and in some places of the central nervous system. Fortunately for us, most neurotransmitters do not change at all—we keep the same numbers of them and keep the ability to make new ones. Some that scientists have found to diminish in aging are the catecholamines, a class of neurotransmitters of which norerinephrine and dopamine are well known. Others, such as acetylcholine and serotonin, diminish only slightly during a lifetime. Catecholamine reduction has been measured in the hypothalamus where so many hormonal releasing factors originate. Thus, some of the hormonal changes observed in aging may be explained.

Changes occur, too, in neurotransmitter metabolism. Some of the enzymes producing the neurotransmitters, one of which is tyrosine hydrozylase which regulates the production of dopamine and norepinephrine, have been found to decrease in activity in the basal ganglia sections of the brain, while another, monoamine oxidase, which inhibits some neurotransmitters, actually increases in quantity with age.

Why is there an aging reduction in the catecholamines? No one knows for sure, but one cause may be arteriosclerosis. If there is a changed quantity of blood reaching the brain with oxygen, the metabolism of neurotransmitters will be affected. Again, a safeguard we can take is regular exercise to keep the blood vessels open. And a diet low in fats with a good balance of vitamins and minerals can surely help. Vitamins and minerals are necessary for our synthesis of the enzymes which, in turn, make the neurotransmitters.

Parkinson's Disease

Parkinson's disease and several similar diseases of the neuromuscular system are believed to be related to reduced metabolism of dopamine and other catecholamine neurotransmitters. Our autonomic nervous system, properly working, has a balance of two types of impulses. One of them "excites," causing movement, and the other "inhibits" or stops movement. Neurotransmitters also function in one or the other of these ways, depending on the tissue they inhabit at the moment. In Parkinson's disease, there seems to be an inability to maintain the balance between excitation and inhibition of the muscles, along with a difficulty in starting movement. The result is jerks and tremors—the hand trem-

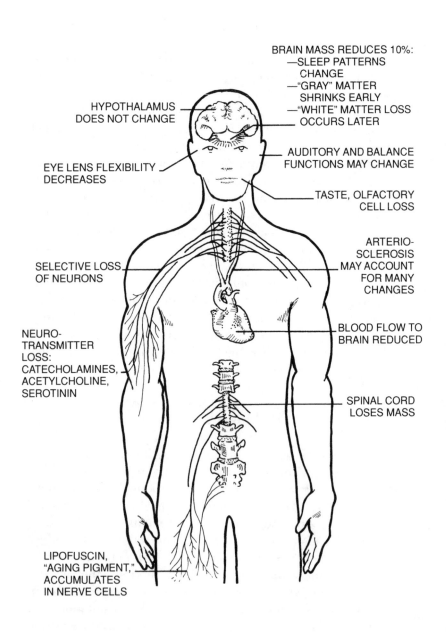

BRAIN MASS REDUCES 10%:
—SLEEP PATTERNS CHANGE
—"GRAY" MATTER SHRINKS EARLY
—"WHITE" MATTER LOSS OCCURS LATER

HYPOTHALAMUS DOES NOT CHANGE

AUDITORY AND BALANCE FUNCTIONS MAY CHANGE

EYE LENS FLEXIBILITY DECREASES

TASTE, OLFACTORY CELL LOSS

ARTERIO-SCLEROSIS MAY ACCOUNT FOR MANY CHANGES

SELECTIVE LOSS OF NEURONS

NEURO-TRANSMITTER LOSS: CATECHOLAMINES, ACETYLCHOLINE, SEROTININ

BLOOD FLOW TO BRAIN REDUCED

SPINAL CORD LOSES MASS

LIPOFUSCIN, "AGING PIGMENT," ACCUMULATES IN NERVE CELLS

Figure 20 The changing central nervous system

bles because the stimulation to inhibit movement is over-whelmed by excitation impulses. The reason that the drug, levodopa, can restore the balance for some people or control the most extreme tremors for others is that it helps our own enzymes make dopamine.

Some interesting experimental studies have shown that L-dopa, as levodopa is usually called, lengthens the lives of laboratory rats of some particular genetic strains. It has even restored the estrous cycles of aging rats but it has shown neither of these results in people. Of other treatments being studied for Parkinson's disease, one of the most promising is a technique for transplanting cells from the adrenal gland to the brain. The cells make the hormones epinephrine and nor-epinephrine which are chemically similar to dopamine. Swedish scientists who have tried the technique on several patients with success in alleviating tremors in some of them are hopeful they will eventually grow dopamine-synthesizing cells in a laboratory for implantation in Parkinson's patients.

Some of our growing knowledge of the disease comes from observations that certain antipsychotic drugs, like lithium carbonate, when given in fairly large quantities, can upset the catecholamine balance, bringing on Parkinson's-like symptoms. A growing number of scientists believe the disease can be caused by ingestion of molecules of certain pesticides. Many victims of an encephalitis epidemic in the United States in the 1920s developed Parkinson's disease twenty or thirty years later. The reason? The encephalitis virus took up residence in the brain, destroying cells in the basal ganglia region, lowering the levels of catecholamines. Later, when the people lost more catecholamines as they aged, their levels were so low that Parkinson's resulted. Now most scientists think that since we make fewer of our own catecholamines when we reach old age, those of us who had low levels to begin with are the likely candidates to show symptoms of Parkinson's. So there is genetic susceptibility to the disease. But the normal reduction of catecholamines due to aging is not great enough in itself to bring on Parkinson's.

Multiple Sclerosis

Multiple sclerosis is an autoimmune disease characterized by destruction of the myelin insulation of nerve cells, destruction which can occur in the brain or in any of the body's nerve cells. It is a disease commonly beginning in the young adult years, more often in women than men. It is marked by sudden onsets of neurological symptoms, such as muscle weakness, lack of coordination, and dimness of vision. Victims experience long periods of being symptom-free, but it is a progressively weakening disease.

Although the cause of multiple sclerosis is not definitely known, the slow virus theory is prominent since measles virus antibodies have been found in the lesions of people with the disease. Scientific knowledge of slow viruses had a grisly genesis. D. C. Gajdusek, a scientisit studying a tribe of cannibals in New Guinea, found in 1957 that kuru, a degenerative disease of the cerebellum with tremors and balance disturbances, passed from the old tribal members to the young. It was a practice of these people to ingest the wisdom of their elders figuratively by literally eating the brains of their deceased relatives. A virus quite similar to the encephalitis variety was being passed to the young people during the funeral feasts. Needless to say, the practice was halted, the incidence of the disease fell strikingly, and Gajdusek won a Nobel prize. Scientists have not yet discovered the mode of transmission of the multiple sclerosis slow virus, if that is truly the cause of the disease.

Our brain and central nervous system have a certain content of fat, primarily the myelin membrane or insulation of neurons, and in the absence of disease our amount of myelin remains rather constant as we age, although the types of lipids used to make up the insulation shift in composition. There have been studies showing that some of the components of young myelin, such as cholesterol and triglycerides, are replaced in later years by different phospholipids. No implication of this shift in fat composition is yet apparent, but it may have something to do with other fats, called lipofuscins—aging pigments which seem to collect in many of the brain's neurons as we age. Lipofuscin is a yellow, granular waste material much like ear wax. It builds up inside many nerve cells over the years and there is no evidence that it is harmful, although it may contribute to reduced protein synthesis since it occupies space in the cell, crowding out other components used in making proteins. But lipofuscin may even be beneficial to us. One theory is that it traps toxic substances in the neurons, keeping them safe from damage.

Hopeful news appeared for multiple sclerosis victims in the late summer 1987, with a report from the Albert Einstein College of Medicine in New York and the Weizmann Institute of Science in Israel. A synthetically-produced substance called COP 1 produced, in a two-year experiment, "clinically important and statistically significant beneficial effects" in at least the early stages of some multiple sclerosis cases.

Senile Dementia and Alzheimer's Disease

Changing position, in the literal sense of postural change, creates changes in blood pressure. When we stand up suddenly after sitting for a time in a chair or even rise up on our elbows from a prone position, the body must adjust its blood pressure regulation. A moment of lightheadedness means that adjustments are underway, reflex actions to dilate the arteries. While hardening of the arteries means more reflex time is needed for blood pressure control in old people, changes in the neurotransmitter levels can add even more time. As we change position, signals from the brain instruct baroreceptors in the aorta and carotid areas to relax the vessels, so the neurotransmitters that help the impulse along have an effect on blood pressure. In studies observing young and old people rapidly changing postural positions, a far greater amount of norepinephrine has been found imme-diately circulating in the young.

Changing position implies much more for us as we age than just blood pressure readjustment upon getting out of bed. When we retire from our accustomed activities of forty years, we have changed our position. Retirement usually means that we have half the income—or less—that we have grown used to having; our position at the bank changes. When our spouse dies or when our friends die, we experience stressful changes of habitual and social position. Remark-ably, our species adapts to changed positions. It is human nature, implying much more than biology, to adjust. But none of our adaptive capacity can help us if we are unfortunate enough to have brain failure, usually called organic brain syndrome. Senile dementia and Alzheimer's disease are the most familiar of these conditions.

"On Golden Pond" by Ernest Thompson touchingly dra-matized our fears of senile dementia. The principal character of the play, 80-year old Norman Thayer, walks into the woods not far from his summer home and, fearfully, realizes that he is lost. He has tramped through these same woods all his life; indeed, he knows them as well as he knows the rooms and hallways of his home, yet on this particular morning, he recognizes not one tree or one path. It is as if he is seeing the surroundings for the first time in his life. He does not know where he is. In Norman's brain, the images he sees do not associate with his memory. All he can remember is how to hurry back to the safety of home. There he tells his wife he fears his mind is fading away.

For Norman, the brain dysfunction was transitory, but it was as real to him as nightmares can be when we wake up, startled, believing for a moment or two we are really experi-encing dreamed events. Senile dementia means the loss of memory, orientation, reasoning, and language ability. But it does not come suddenly one summer morning in the woods. The most common form of senile dementia, Alzheimer's dis-ease, has a quite slow and progressive onset. People with

Alzheimer's can eventually lose all their personal habits, including their hygiene, and then require fulltime nursing care. Two new drugs, naloxone and physostigmine, are being used with limited success to reverse some symptoms. Scientists believe, though, that drug therapy will one day be able to control most senile dementia disorders.

Norman's experience in "On Golden Pond" was not senile dementia, but a temporary memory loss (most probably due to imbalances in neurotransmitter metabolism). His nerve impulses were sidetracked at the synapses and not enough of them were getting through for him to conjure up associations for memory. Senile dementia's causes, on the other hand, are still matters of speculation. Arteriosclerosis is thought to be a contributing cause, but also suspected are slow viruses, autoimmunity, genetic error, tangled nerve cell filaments, senile plaques, and even aluminum—if too much of this mineral finds its way into the brain. Traces of aluminum have been found in the brains of people who had Alzheimer's disease when they died. It is present in drinking water and most anti-perspirants; it is added to many of our foods and drugs, such as processed cheese, antacids, and buffered aspirin; and, of course, a little rubs off from cans in which soft drinks are sold.

Neuronal loss, dendritic loss, and faulty neurotransmitters cannot be the sole causes of Alzheimer's disease; they are a part of normal aging yet less than five percent of people over 65 have any type of organic brain syndrome. It may be that all of these factors working together bring on brain disorders. Alzheimer's disease, if this is true, is caused by an accumulation of factors. Its victims have some or all of the factors in more advanced states than normal elderly people do. The normal brain loses about ten percent of its weight by age 80; in senile dementia, about another ten percent is lost. Autopsies of the brains of people with Alzheimer's disease have shown neuronal loss at the base of the brain, an area important for cholinergic neurotransmitters, especially acetylcholine. It is this neurotransmitter which is necessary for mediating nerve impulses dealing with memory function. This finding suggests that drug therapy might prove effective for Alzheimer's, for instance, the administration of a drug to help the body produce acetylcholine, just as L-dopa aids Parkinson's victims in restoring dopamine levels. So far, though, a safe and effective drug remains elusive, although some experiments with a new drug called THA have shown hopeful results. Purified lecithin appears promising to some researchers—the body breaks down lecithin to form choline.

Neurofibrillary tangles and senile plaques are apparently also part of the aging process, since they are seen in microscopic examinations of normal, elderly brains. One area where the tangles are found in most old people is the hippocampal cortex, a part of the brain involved with the memory process. In people with Alzheimer's disease, however, tangles and plaques are found in much larger numbers. Neurons are composed of two fibers or filaments of protein—tubulin and filarin. When these filaments twist around each other, they become a neurofibrillary tangle and they lose their proper function. What causes them to twist together?

Stanley R. Prusiner of the University of California, San Francisco, School of Medicine has identified an infectious agent he calls a "prion" in the brains of sheep with the fatal disease, scrapie. There is a possibility the prion which, unlike a virus, has neither DNA nor RNA, is associated with Alzheimer's. Scientists think that perhaps a virus or a prion causes a genetic error, resulting in instructions for the creation of a protein different from tubulin and filarin. Since they are found in many persons over 60, another theory has it that neurofibrillary tangles are instruments of the biological clock, a naturally occurring mechanism planned for the purpose of weakening the individual who will deteriorate and die.

Senile or neuritic plaques are also found in the brains of most elderly people, but they are found in large numbers in people who have senile dementia. They appear to be collections of antibody-like material and cellular wastes from mitochrondrial metabolic processes. As in multiple sclerosis, it is thought that autoimmunity may be a factor in creating neuritic plaques. They occur not only in the brain but also in other nerves of the body and are accompanied by a loss of myelin insulation.

Depression

If organic brain syndrome has been found not to be an inevitable corollary of old age, neither is it the most common mental disorder of the elderly. That all old people become mentally senile is part of society's longstanding and totally incorrect attitude of ageism. If our elderly parent is forgetful, we tend to say, "Oh, she's getting senile." In actuality, Mother may have always been slightly forgetful. We assign stereotypical mental illness to old people when illness does not even exist or when, in actuality, they may be confused or depressed because of a physical ailment or too much drug-medicine. Old age, in itself, does not bring mental illness; a grumpy old person most likely was a grumpy young person. Sudden symptoms of mental illness are usually signs of a problem that can be treated. Such symptoms may be caused by a change in blood pressure pills or a combination of tranquilizers and aspirin. That the real causes of so much mental depression in old people go untreated, and so often old people are pronounced senile and packed away into isolation, is a sad indictment of our society's ignorance in geriatric medicine. Of the five percent of elderly people whose conditions are diagnosed as senile dementia, almost one-third are really suffering from physical causes such as ailments of the kidney, liver, or heart; from treatable psychiatric disorders; or from the effects of drug-medicine. Many old people take medicine for their blood pressure or cardiac arrhythmias. Inderal, digitalis, and L-dopa (the drug used for Parkinson's disease) are known to cause depression. So do many antibiotics used for treating pulmonary infections.

In fact, the most common psychiatric problem in elderly people is depression and close behind is hypochondriasis. It is no wonder. Our culture has equated growing old with depression and physical infirmity. So when we reach old age, we expect to be depressed—just as we expect to be sick. We are conditioned to look on each physical change of aging as an ailment. Excluded from the workplace, social life vastly reduced, income cut in half, talents and experience gone to waste, our elderly are buried before their death. In what contrast Western society stands to the cannibals of New Guinea who until the last few years ate the brains of their old relatives innocently wanting to reap their wisdom. We isolate our elderly, shamefully allowing their wisdom to wither away with their spirits, minds, and bodies. The result: loneliness for our old people, no exercise, poor nutrition, lack of a purpose for living, real and imagined illnesses, and, making everything even worse, overmedication. We engender physical and mental depression in our old people. A shocking statistic: One-fourth of those who commit suicide in the United States are over 65 years old.

Depression may, of course, be organic; that is, it may have a biological cause of its own. The combination of changes in the endocrine and nervous systems in old age depresses or slows some of the body's physical activity. Many hormones operate at reduced levels along with reductions in neurons and neurotransmitters. If this brings on depressed physical activity, it more than likely can bring on depressed mental activity. But such depression can be treated and should be treated. Old people respond to psychiatric treatment just as young people do.

Neither reduced intellectual capacity nor pessimism are biological changes of aging; they are cultural changes of aging. And just as we make adjustments for our biological changes, we can make adjustments in our incorrect, behind-the-times attitudes about growing old. Good physical health requires good mental health and vice versa. No less than we need regular, vigorous exercise for the body, we need to make a habit of vigorous mental exercise. We need to continue our intellectual interests or develop new ones. Most of all, we need to throw away our defeatist attitude about aging. Pessimism is a hindrance, it is never of any worthwhile use. Indeed, it is harmful since it is stressful. Changing a position of pessimism for a hopeful attitude of good health—mental and physical—is a positive aging adjustment. Just like regular, vigorous, physical exercise, it takes a period of determination before it becomes an enjoyable routine.

Chapter 12

Straight Talk About Life and Death

Ageism and the fear of aging conspire to keep the biological mysteries of our changing bodies locked away from human knowledge. Aging is like the news channel on television— why watch it when a switch of the knob tunes in fantasy scenes of youth, sexual desire fulfilled, glamor and materialism, or, most often, advertisements of hokum products which promise that youth and glamor can be ours? Aging is a fact of life, and cannot be reversed by wishful thinking. Its worrisome effects, however, may be minimized by a lifelong enjoyment of regular exercise, a regimen of good and balanced nutrition, and a habit of positive thinking.

As we grow older, we need to stay attuned to the changes taking place in our bodies—changes that most likely will mean we must adjust our activity level. Growing old successfully means making positive adjustments and taking up new activities which suit the requirements of older age. Aging ballet dancers who discover with dismay that they cannot leap halfway across a stage make a positive adjustment when they become teachers. They, as elders, pass on their wisdom and experience to young members of their profession. In the same way, an Olympic swimmer ages successfully when he becomes the coach of a swim team. The choices are the same for us all, no matter what we have made of our youth and middle age: We may choose a sedentary life; we may build a wall around us and withdraw from life; or we can take control of our changing lives and adapt them to new activities, new experiences.

The secret of successful aging presents itself at each stage of our lives. It really is no secret for it is so obvious: Making the most of youth, the young adult years, middle age, and then old age is to create experiences which remain with us throughout life. Experiences become the past, but they live on in the present through memory and subconscious motivations. This storehouse of experiences offers us the satisfaction of a life well-lived. Contentment with the way we have lived is a pleasure we can hardly know when we are young. It is the peace of mind we may look forward to experiencing before we die.

Death, like aging, is a fact of life. Death is inherent in our design; the primary forces behind our aging, the forces of genetics, the environment, and evolution, influence our lives in the same pattern and they all play a part in seeing to it that we age and then die. The molecule of DNA that we inherit from our parents contains our biological clock, our potential for a long, healthy life or our potential for susceptibility to disease with an early death. Wear and tear from the world around us, the environment in which we live and the manner in which we live, can guide or misguide our genetic inheritance. As human beings we are, every one of us, not only masterworks of evolution's progression, but also individual members of an ever-changing species, one that is ever more adaptable to a changing world. It is Mother Nature's plan that we die to make room for those who will follow. Evolution thus makes us eternal, if only by the passage of DNA from generation to generation. Unlike our ancestors, we no longer live in trees and caves, but rather in comfort-controlled, computer-monitored home environments. We continue to be an adaptable species. How are we more adaptable than we were fifty years ago? We have developed the technology for leaving our world and colonizing another planet—if we can find one that is suitable. Evolutionary adaptability comes through improvements of our intellectual powers no less than through improvements of physical vigor. Biological knowledge of the aging process allows us to adapt further by taking control of some of the mechanisms heretofore directing our aging as if we were string puppets.

Aging and death are facts of life, but how we age and how we die are not at all certain. Each person ages at a unique rate depending on his genes and his environment, and each person eventually dies from a disease—unless accident gets him first. There is really no such thing as death from "old age," although we would like to think so. It is pathology, not old age, that stops life. Pathology—whether from traumatic accident, infectious agent, or faulty cellular regulation—causes death either when the heart and lungs stop or when the brain stops.

Death, like religion and politics, involves faith and endless questioning. There is not much we can know about death and so there is much to fear about it. Mankind has always feared death, but the form of our fear changes with the times and with our circumstances. Fear of a violent death is not prevalent today although it certainly was the main fear for very early man, sharing as he did an environment with wild beasts of other species much larger than he was. Later, the Egyptians feared that grave-robbers would interfere with the difficult journey of their after-life and so they protected their dead bodies with elaborate tombs and sophisticated embalming techniques. Downplaying all that and casting aside any attempt to preserve the body, the Greeks feared that they would die before they had the opportunity to learn all of life's truths; they hoped for heaven on earth. Throughout most Judaeo-Christian history, the fear has been of what comes after death. The concept of heaven after death continues to be a reassuring and comforting belief for the dying. What we fear most today is the dying process, the pain and the suffering that come before death, for we have begun to prolong unhealthy lives. Years ago, people usually died quickly from acute diseases; nowadays, death can be a long, drawn-out process of degeneration—months and years of dependence upon technological means, even though a person's enjoyment of life has died. Bernard Towers, co-director of the UCLA Program in Medicine, Law, and Human Values which has sponsored many public forums on the subject of death in the last few years, points out that the ancient practices of embalming and cremation came back in vogue a few hundred years ago when people feared being pronounced dead and then waking up to find they had been buried. Today, Towers says, our main fear is that we will be kept alive by means of medical machinery longer than we want to be—longer than what is dignified.

People want to die with their dignity intact. Spending your final months or years intubated for nutrition that you cannot enjoy, suffering from hip ulcers or bed sores because you cannot physically rise, watching your life savings transfer to the hospitals' corporate board—this is not a dignified end to a human life. We do not have to choose this sort of death.

Pulling the Plug

You wouldn't think that the definition of death is problematic, but we still have disagreement in our society in deciding when someone is dead. Until the 1980s, half of the states in the United States said in their legal statutes that the stopping of the heart and lungs—cardiopulmonary arrest—constitutes death. The other half held that death occurs only when the brain stops. Because medical technology has made it possible to keep a person alive who would die without medical intervention such as the ventilator, intravenous feeding, or hydration by intubaton, the need for a consistent definition of death has gained importance. In 1981, the Uniform Determination of Death Act was developed by a Presidential commission in collaboration with the American Medical Association and the American Bar Association. It recommended an either/or approach: A person is dead when he has sustained either "irreversible cessation of circulatory and respiratory functions, or irreversible cessation of all functions of the entire brain, including the brain stem."

The commission also confronted a more difficult question: When may doctors withhold extraordinary medical measures and allow patients with terminal illnesses to die? "Deciding to Forego Life-Sustaining Treatment," the 1983 report of the commissioners, says that people have the right, generally, to refuse such care (also called heroic measures) and to die if they prefer. Doctors, the report said, "should try to enhance patients' understanding of the available treatment options." But what about people who are unconscious or so ill they cannot make their own decisions? The commission advised reliance on the judgment of physicians and family members and suggested that hospitals form ethics committees made up not only of physicians and hospital employees, but also of social workers, church, and lay people, to make decisions for those who cannot. The problem is that committees of this sort are not always readily convenable when the decisions are needed. The physician, as he always has been, is still our bottom-line decision-maker and our legal-minded society has made him nervous and reluctant to "pull the plug"—even in the most obviously terminal circumstances.

The hesitancy is understandable. Keeping people alive—prolonging life—is the physician's primary job and at times in history he could lose his own head if the patient who died was a pharoah or a king. More recently, the physician's plight is not so dire; he has merely been a defendant in expensive malpractice lawsuits. He must pay ever-increasing insurance premiums for such an eventuality. The dilemma is compounded since physicians also believe their job is to relieve suffering—an obligation that can sometimes run counter to the other task of prolonging life. Sometimes the best way to relieve suffering is *not* to prolong life.

Meanwhile, the physician must pay close attention to the courts' rulings, rulings which attempt to monitor advances in medicine. Intravenous feeding and intubation are not qualitatively different from the respirator as means of prolonging life, according to the New Jersey Supreme Court's recent decision, "In the Matter of Claire C. Conroy," which further argued that a valid proxy has the legal right to decide when withholding is appropriate for a terminally ill person who cannot decide for himself.

The sort of new medical machinery that technology keeps developing costs enormous sums of money and is a principal reason why health care continues to become more expensive. Can we as a society afford such increasingly costly medical treatment? The way our medical system operates now allows the rich an advantage. Their lives can be extended by their own money in private hospitals while people with limited means are dumped (a word being used by the medical establishment) to publicly-funded hospitals. County, city, and state hospitals thus become more and more pinched in the pursestrings in an effort to provide equitable care. The Presidential commission attacked this problem, too, and concluded that . . . "health care institutions may justifiably restrict the availability of certain options in order to use limited resources more effectively or to enhance equity in allocating them." This means more decisions must be made by physicians and committees, by government agencies and the court system. The real problem is that our society values equal opportunity for everyone, but we are realizing that we cannot afford to make the new marvels of medical technology available to everyone, our economic state of affairs being what they are. We would like to make medical care equitable, but we cannot pay for it. Just maintaining the partial payments systems such as Medicare strains society's means. If we want a truly equitable system then someone, it appears, must make decisions about rationing certain care. And who will make those decisions?

Hospital, Hospice, or Home?

In the last few decades, the ways we die have changed along with our increased longevity. At the turn of the century, when average life expectancy was 47, the leading causes of death were infectious diseases such as pneumonia, tuberculosis, influenza, and gastroenteritis. Many child-bearing women died because of complications during pregnancy. Advances in medicine, surgery, and sanitation changed the picture so that we now survive our bouts with infections and we die later, and on the average, at ages in the mid-seventies, from heart disease, cancer, cerebrovascular disease, or trauma—the latter including accidents, homicides, and suicides. These four causes account for about seventy-five percent of the two million deaths in the United States each year.

Where we die has also changed dramatically in our century. Until the middle of the twentieth century, people usually died at home or on the battlefield. But now, it is estimated, about eighty percent of deaths take place in hospitals or in nursing homes. Dying people are there, of course, because that is where the physicians and medical technology are. Since physicians rarely make housecalls today, you have to go to them in the hospitals. Another reason why people die in hospitals is because they do not want their families to share in their suffering. "I don't want to be a burden" or "The children shouldn't have to worry about me" are the common sentiments expressed. Unfortunately, this attitude contributes to our fear of death. By removing death from sight, we forget that it is a fact of life.

Dying in a hospital is criticized for its institutional, impersonal setting and because often, although life is prolonged, irreversible illnesses and suffering are prolonged in the process. Changes, though, have begun. A recent trend is the visiting nurse who provides care at the patient's home and teaches family members to provide care. It is now common to have tube feeding and intravenous food and drug administration in the home. A few years ago, intravenous therapy was considered a hospital procedure only.

The hospice, an alternative to both home and an institutional setting for death, was a widely-praised experiment in the Seventies that has caught on. Such places, sometimes but not always under the auspices of a hospital, provide a home-like setting for terminally-ill people. No heroic measures are taken to prolong life in a hospice, but much is done to relieve suffering. So often in our society no preparations are made for death—important preparations like financial arrangements and estate inheritance—because we tend to deny that the end is so near. Family members are often unprepared for the stress and psychological readjustment that come with the death of a loved one. Talking about death and actively preparing for it by settling one's affairs are encouraged in hospices. And it is not just the dying patient who talks, but also his family members. Perhaps a fundamental advantage of the hospice is that patients and their families realistically accept that death is near. Thus, the hospice serves a need of the dying and of the living. There are other differences between hospices and hospitals. A hospice needs to be well-staffed, not just in numbers of nurses, but in caring, compassionate nurses who have had special training. Hospices provide space for family members to stay overnight and even to cook meals for their dying relatives. Homecooking in lieu of hospital food is, decidedly, a step forward in making death less fearsome and more comfortable.

Hospices are expensive and were largely financed by charitable means until 1982, when federal legislation extended Medicare reimbursements to patients in them. Like all legislation striving for equitability, Medicare hospice reimbursement is restricted to certain patients, certain diseases, and certain prognoses such as "six months," so it goes nowhere near making a comfortable death available to everyone. Our society is not yet ready to commit its money to making death less fearsome and more comfortable. Besides, hospices do not make money. Matthew Conolly, Professor of Medicine and Pharmacology at UCLA, makes a point when he says, "We choose to spend fifteen million dollars on (producing) one soft-drink commercial, but we're too selfish to provide hospice care." Other critics of the legislation foresee that under Medicare, the hospice will go the way of the nursing home industry—big business. The road could easily lead to impersonal, institution-like death homes. Who needs those?

Choices

We are living, aging, and dying in a time when more and more choices are open to us. The hospice is an alternative to lives of disease and discomfort extended by medical machinery. Death is discussed instead of ignored. We may write "living wills" and designate a family member or friend to make decisions for us if we become too sick to do so. We can choose to die by suicide which is no longer against the law in most places, although "assisted suicide" (help in dying from family, friend, or physician) continues to be a crime for the helper even though judges are often lenient when the case is obviously a merciful death. Choices affecting living and aging abound. The knowledge we are gaining about genetics is still in its primitive stage, but already it is raising questions and options that we human beings have hardly thought about, so busy have we been thus far in our history with survival questions: feeding ourselves, tribal and national boundaries, and war. Besides those still troublesome questions, we now have others. Are we prepared to know, for instance, what disease will cause our death twenty years from now? Genetics gives us the potential for that knowledge. Do we want to know if our particular disease or death will occur in our forties, or in our fifties, or in our sixties? Would we want to know we have a thirty percent probability of developing osteoporosis at age 55 or a twenty-six percent probability of cancer at 75? Do we want to know this? It is something we need to think about, because such knowledge will probably be available to us sooner than we think. Already, such diseases as Huntington's chorea, sickle cell anemia, Tay-Sachs disease, and Down's syndrome are reliably predicted *in utero*. In the future, babies may be "genotyped" at birth—a genetic operation in which a biopsied cell sample can be run through a computer which will print out a whole life "program" showing disease tendencies, expected cause of death, and even time of death. The procedure might be called genetic fortune-telling (or palm reading, if the cell sample comes from the infant's palm). The advantage of knowing this information is that preventive action could be taken to forestall the onset of the disease, or to lessen its effects. If you know you have a predisposition to lung cancer you certainly will not smoke cigarettes. If you know you have the genetic marker for hypercholesterolemia you will start an exercise program as soon as you can walk.

What about not knowing? Do we have the right *not* to know our disease potential or when we may die? If our lives are mapped out for us in advance, at least from a physical point of view, will we undergo a fundamental psychological change? We human beings have always lived in the dark with respect to our personal futures. We make the basic decisions in our lives, decisions about education, careers, and whom we will share our lives with, under the assumption that we will live about 75 years. Might those decisions be different if we knew in advance that we have an eighty percent chance of leukemia by the time we reach 35? The answer depends on "if's." If there is a way to stop cancer, it certainly is to our advantage to know in advance about our own susceptibility. But if there is no cure, what kind of day-to-day life would it be for a 20-year old who carries around a genetic print-out that stops at 35?

Questions like these are no longer fanciful. Scientists are deciphering genetic codes and unravelling puzzles for us. But it is we, not the scientists, who will have to decide what to do with the knowledge of genetics or, at least, we need to decide who should make the decisions. Should it be the scientists? Should it be our elected leaders? Should it be committees? Who will sit on the committees? Who will appoint them? The questions must be addressed.

And if we could discover a way to stop aging. What do we mean when we make such a wish? Do we really want immortality? Do we want to live two hundred years? A hundred and fifty? Or do we want to change the aging process in ways to let us maintain a particular age? If so, what age? Some people think 35 is a good age. Some believe 25 is better and, of course, some think 50 is the best of all. At any rate, there is always accident. We will never be immortal simply because accident will get us sooner or later. If pathology passes us by completely, we will one day be on one of those airplanes that come down or in an automobile crash. We just might put an end to disease but we will never be able to completely protect ourselves from accidents.

With our new knowledge about disease and biological aging, more and more people are opting for lives of good health, carefully planning their diet and exercise routines just as carefully as they plan their careers, and just as carefully as they plan how to minimize the effects of stress. With better health in our older years, retirement from careers is quickly becoming less mandatory, more optional for many people. Why quit working if we like to work? Conversely, why not? If we spend our adult lives in unrewarding tedious toil, retirement is something to look forward to.

A new crop of doomsayers has emerged in the last few years, speaking and writing and generally spreading alarm that in the near future young adults will have to give larger and larger portions of their earnings to care for a swelling tide of the old and chronically disabled. This is the old picture of ageism—based on a bizarre assumption that young people have such a lack of respect for older people that they do not want to share in society's expense of providing a minimal existence for them. Those now spreading the alarm enjoy using statistics, demographic tables, and charts to show the multiplying numbers of elderly people in the United States. Statistical interpretations of where society is going, however, are not taking other changes into consideration. Nor can anyone truly predict what lies in the future, especially when society's changing attitudes are considered. By dwelling on numbers and ignoring the changing picture of overall health in people, the statisticians are only planting age prejudice in young people. With interpretations such as "One working person will have to pay taxes to support three retired people," they engender resentment toward elderly people. With declarations like "Health care costs will be such a severe strain on society that medical care will need to be rationed in favor of the young," they give everyone a fear of aging. Statistics are necessary for predicting trends and for preparing for the future, but editorializing about what people's attitudes will be is wrong. It is ageism in its roots.

From time to time, graduate students in gerontology conduct public polls and report that there are signs of more positive attitudes toward old age. The trouble is, they present a list of human conditions such as cancer, alcoholism, mental illness, criminal behavior—and old age—and then ask their respondents to rank the list from one to ten. Then they publish their findings in theses or journals and point out with satisfaction that old age comes out high on the list. The interpretation: The public views being elderly as slightly more desirable than being an ex-convict. Aren't such polls employing ageism as their premise?

Why Not Be Hopeful?

There was a time not long ago when physicians did not tell patients they had cancer. The feeling was to spare a dying person the knowledge that he was dying. Brutal honesty is the watchword today, of course. Physicians inform their patients that statistics show that ninety-nine out of a hundred people with such-and-such a disease will die. Your chance is one out of a hundred, they say. What has happened is that the useful tool of statistics has been turned into a manner of stressing the negative. The motivation for not telling a patient he has a terminal disease was that he'd not lose hope. But now hope must struggle out from underneath a mountain of statistical despair. Instead of one chance in a hundred, why don't physicians tell patients they *have* a chance? An individual chance?

We need to plan for our changing society—there is no question about that. But it is quite questionable to assume that old is the same as disabled or that old age necessarily must be a burden on the young. It is quite questionable to assume that fifty million people over age 75 will be people who depend on other people. These are unfounded fears. The reason our numbers of elderly people are multiplying these days is because we are growing old in good health—statistically and individually. Our society is making possible a longer period of youth, a longer period of middle age, and a longer period of old age. Why can't we assume that such will continue to be the case? It could be that a downward trend in chronic, degenerative disease in the elderly, with an increase in acute diseases, will relieve some of the present need for long-term health care. The present interest in physical fitness will certainly change the proportions of chronically ill elderly people. You cannot predict, simply because a certain proportion of old people required round-the-clock nursing care in 1970, that the proportion will be the same in the year 2020. Better health care because of medical advances and better health because of changing habits of people as they are aging can likely mean that by the year 2020, a smaller proportion of elderly people will be chronically sick. After all, most present-day old people never thought of going to a gym when they were young adults or jogging a half-hour every morning.

Why not be hopeful that our old age will be a time of comfort and of good health? Being hopeful promotes good health, while being fearful is to stress the body's resources. Why not be hopeful that science will continue to find causes and cures for the chronic, degenerative diseases of old age? And why not be hopeful that as we age we will see adjustments in society's priorities? The portion of all our resources going into scientific research and health care is far smaller than what we spend perpetuating enmity throughout our world. "Defense" is our euphemistic reason for this. Current priorities direct disproportionate quantities of our money and intellectual talents toward guarding the borders between peoples, an illustration of how little we have advanced from our tribal past. We have made stupendous advances in technological ways but, sadly, we still are struggling to attain a world civilization of trust and brotherhood. Why not be hopeful that we will soon change our priorities and put a stop to this wasted drain of our resources? Instead of billions of dollars for weapons of disease and death, why not use the money to make our world more comfortable for us all? Why isn't anti-carcinogen research a higher priority with us than weapons that destroy life? Why do we channel our resources toward endangering life and health rather than improving them? It is a matter of choice.

The ways we age are shaped by choices as well as by biology. René DuBos, a scientifically-trained humanist, was 80 years old when he wrote his optimistic *Celebrations of Life,* which argued that what distinguishes us human beings from most other species of life on earth is that we "can choose among several possible courses of action, thus transcending the constraints of biological determinism through . . . free will." The choices for taking control of our own aging are more available to us today than at any time in history. We have hard and fast evidence that exercise eases the adjustments of aging bodies. The specific amount of exercise for each of us remains mostly a matter of choice. In the developed world, at least, we have the good fortune to be able to choose a balanced, moderate diet. We may look forward to more and better control of health through science and medicine. We also may choose the positive mental activity of keeping good health uppermost in our thoughts.

A wise choice we can make is to banish from our thoughts the fear of aging. Growing old should not be a time of dread and apprehension. We should anticipate it, rather, as the time in our lives when we may add the final layers of our development as human beings. We never lose our youth—it is there, still a part of us, as memory and as guiding influence.

If we build upon it, youth can deepen and broaden into maturity, but we retain it, just as all our experiences become part of what we are. Sights and smells and tastes and tunes stimulate memories within our neuronal network, reminding us that what we are is what we were, and what we are is what we will become. We don't lose anything; as we age we have only to gain.

The biological miracles which created us have given us all the ages of life—child, teen, young adult, middle age, and old age. It is up to us whether we choose to make the most of each. Going from one stage to the next, perhaps the most important adjustment we can make as we age and change is to realize that the importance of life is not longevity, but how life is lived and enjoyed and appreciated. What is aging if not the accumulation of experience? Aging is developing and growing in knowledge and wisdom. Mother Nature gave us our instinctive urge toward youthful beauty so that we would reproduce ourselves. Ah, but there's another beauty that is only discerned by living and aging. Like a taste for the good things, the beauty of aging is an acquired taste. What an exciting feeling it is to wake up with the sunrise, healthy and eager to be productive. There is no substitute.

Is it long life we want or is it contentment with the life we have lived?

Bibliography

Abram, M.B. Chairman: *Deciding to Forego Life-Sustaining Treatment.* Washington, D.C.: U.S. Government Printing Office, 1983, 83-600503.

Aloia, J.L. *et al:* Prevention of Involutional Bone Loss by Exercise. *Annals of Internal Medicine,* 89: 356–358, 1978.

Ames, B.N.: Dietary Carcinogens and Anticarcinogens. *Science,* 221: 1256–1264, 1983.

Arntzenius, A.C. *et al:* Diet, Lipoproteins, and the Progression of Coronary Atherosclerosis. *New England Journal of Medicine,* 312: 805–811, 1985.

Behnke, J.A., Finch, C.E., & Moment, G.B. (Eds.): *The Biology of Aging.* New York: Plenum, 1978.

Beljan, J.R. *et al:* Dementia (report by the Council on Scientific Affairs of the American Medical Association). *Journal of the American Medical Association,* 256: 2234–2238, 1986.

Bell, E., Marek, L.F., Levinstone, D.S., Merrill, C., Sher, S., Young, I.T., & Eden, M.: Loss of Division Potential in vitro: Aging or Differentiation? *Science,* 202: 1158–1163, 1978.

Bennett, W.I. (Ed.): *The Harvard Medical School Health Letter,* IX: 3–4, 1983.

Bergsma, D. & Harrison, D.E.: *Genetic Effects on Aging.* New York: Liss, 1978.

Bishop, J.M.: Oncogenes. *Scientific American,* 246: 81–92, 1982.

Bornstein, M.B. *et al.:* A Pilot Trial of COP 1 in Exacerbating-Remitting Multiple Sclerosis. *New England Journal of Medicine.* 317: 408–414, 1987.

Braithwaite, R.W. & Lee, A.K.: A mammalian example of semelparity. *The American Naturalist,* 113: 151–155, 1979.

Brill, W.J.: Safety Concerns and Genetic Engineering in Agriculture. *Science,* 227: 381–384, 1985.

Brown, M.S. & Goldstein, J.L.: How LDL Receptors Influence Cholesterol and Atherosclerosis. *Scientific American,* 251(5): 58–66, 1984.

Brown, W.T., Epstein, J., & Little, J.B.: Progeria cells are stimulated to repair DNA by cocultivation with normal cells. *Experimental Cells Research,* 97: 291–296, 1976.

Buckley, W.F.: Reflections on Growing Older. *Modern Maturity,* April–May, 1984, pp. 45–46.

Butler, R.N.: Breaking images: The media and aging. *Columbia Journalism Monograph,* No. 3, New York: Columbia University Press, 1979, pp. 1–11.

Butler, R.N.: 2020 Vision: A Look at the Next Century. *Modern Maturity,* April–May, 1984, pp. 48–49.

Butler, R.N.: *Why Survive? Being Old in America.* New York: Harper and Row, 1975.

Cherkin, A., Finch, C.E., Kharasch, N., Makinodan, T., Scott, F.L., & Strehler, B.L. (Eds.): *Physiology and Cell Biology of Aging.* New York: Raven, 1979.

Council on Scientific Affairs, American Medical Association: Vitamin Preparations as Dietary Supplements and as Therapeutic Agents. *Journal of the American Medical Association*. 257: 1929–1936, 1987.

Cox, H.: *Later Life: The Realities of Aging*. Englewood Cliffs: Prentice-Hall, 1984.

Cristofalo, V.J. & Rosner, B.A.: Modulation of Cell Proliferation and Senescence of WI-38 Cells by Hydrocortisone. *Federation Proceedings*, 38: 1851–1856, 1979.

Cousins, N.: *Anatomy of an Illness as Perceived by the Patient*. New York: W.W. Norton, 1979.

Cousins, N.: *The Healing Heart: Antidotes to Panic and Helplessness*. New York: W.W. Norton, 1983.

Cutler, R.G.: The dysdifferentiative hypothesis of mammalian aging and longevity. In *The Aging Brain: Cellular and Molecular Mechanisms of Aging in the Nervous System*. E. Giacobini *et al.* (Eds.), Chapt. 1. New York: Raven, 1982, pp. 1–19.

DeBusk, F.L.: The Hutchinson-Gilford Progeria Syndrome. *The Journal of Pediatrics*, 80: 697–724, 1972.

Denckla, W.D.: A Time to Die. *Life Sciences*, 16: 31–44, 1975.

Doty, R.L. *et al:* Smell Identification Ability: Changes with Age. *Science*, 226: 1441–1443, 1984.

Dunant, Y. & Israel, M.: The Release of Acetylcholine. *Scientific American*, 252(4): 58–66, 1985.

Edelson, R.L. & Fink, J.M.: The Immunologic Function of Skin. *Scientific American*, 252(6): 46–55, 1985.

Engelhardt, H.T. (Ed.): Patient as Person in Life and Death. *Journal of Medicine and Philosophy*, Vol. 9, 1984.

Ettinger, R.L. & Beck, J.D.: The New Elderly: What Can the Dental Profession Expect? *Geriatric Dentistry*, 2: 62–69, 1982.

Fernandes, G., Yunis, E.J., & Good, R.A.: Influence of diet on survival of mice. *Proceedings of the National Academy of Science*, USA, 73: 1279–1283, 1976.

Finch, C.E. & Hayflick, L. (Eds.): *Handbook of the Biology of Aging*. New York: Van Nostrand Reinhold, 1977.

Finch, C.E. & Schneider, E.L. (Eds.): *Handbook of the Biology of Aging*. 2nd Ed. New York: Van Nostrand Reinhold, 1984.

Florini, J.R. (Ed.): *CRC Handbook of Biochemistry of Aging*. Boca Raton: CRC Press, 1981.

Florini, J.R. *et al:* Somatomedin-C levels in Healthy Young and Old Men: Relationship to Peak and 24-Hour Integrated Levels of Growth Hormone. *Journal of Gerontology*, 40: 2–8, 1985.

Galbraith, J.K.: America's Changing Work Ethic. *Modern Maturity*, April–May, 1984, pp. 47–48.

Goldstein, S.: Human genetic disorders that feature premature onset and accelerated progression of biological aging. In *Genetics of Aging*. Schneider, E.L. (Ed.), Chapt. 7, New York: Plenum, 1978, pp. 171–224.

Good, R.A., Fernandes, G., & West, A.: Nutrition, Immunologic Aging, and Disease. In *Aging and Immunity*. S.K. Singhal *et al* (Eds.): New York: Elsevier/North Holland, 1979, pp. 141–164.

Greenblatt, R.B. (Ed.): *Geriatric Endocrinology*. New York: Raven, 1978.

Greenberg, E.R. *et al:* Breast Cancer in Mothers Given Diethylstilbestrol in Pregnancy. *New England Journal of Medicine*, 311: 1393–1398, 1984.

Griffith, H.W.: *Complete Guide to Prescription and Non-Prescription Drugs*. Tucson: H.P. Books. 1985.

Hacher, A.: Welfare, The Future of an Illusion. *New York Review of Books*, Feb. 28, 1985, pp. 37–43.

Hayflick, L.: The cell biology of human aging. *Scientific American*, 242(1): 58–65, 1980.

Helfman, P.M. & Badda. J.L.: Aspartic Acid Racemization in Tooth Enamel from Living Humans. *Proceedings of the National Academy of Science*, USA, 72: 2891–2894, 1975.

Hsu, J.M. & Davis, R.L.: *Handbook of Geriatric Nutrition*. Park Ridge, N.J.: Noyes, 1981.

Johansen, K.: Aneurysms. *Scientific American*, 247(1): 110–125, 1982.

Kane, R.L., Solomon, D.H., Beck, J.C., Keeler, E.B., & Kane, R.A.: *Geriatrics in the United States*. Lexington, MA.: D.C. Heath, 1981.

Klein, J.: *Immunology: The Science of Self-Nonself Discrimination*. New York: John Wiley & Sons, 1982.

Klemmack, D.L. & Roff, L.L.: Fear of Personal Aging and Subjective Well-Being in Later Life. *Journal of Gerontology,* 39: 756–758, 1984.

Kolata, G.B.: Testing for Cancer Risk. *Science,* 207: 967–969, 1980.

Kovar, M.G.: Health of the elderly and the use of health services. *Public Health Reports,* 92: 9–19, 1977.

Kromhout, D., Bosschieter, E., & Coulander, C.: The Inverse Relation Between Fish Consumption and 20-Year Mortality from Coronary Heart Disease. *New England Journal of Medicine,* 312: 1205–1209, 1985.

Kushi, L.H. *et al:* Diet and 20-Year Mortality from Coronary Heart Disease. *New England Journal of Medicine,* 312: 811–818, 1985.

Lakatua, D.J. *et al:* Circadian Endocrine Time Structure in Humans Above 80 Years of Age. *Journal of Gerontology,* 39: 658–665, 1984.

Lauter, H.: What Do We Know about Alzheimer's Disease Today? *Danish Medical Bulletin,* 30(1): 1–15, 1985.

Lesnoff-Caravaglia, G. (Ed.): *Health Care of the Elderly.* New York: Human Sciences, 1980.

Makinodan, T. & Yunis, E. (Eds.): *Immunology and Aging.* New York: Plenum, 1977.

Martin, W.C. & Wilson, A.J.E. (Eds.): *Aging and Total Health.* St. Petersburg: Eckerd College, 1976.

Marx, J.L.: The Immune System "Belongs in the Body." *Science,* 227: 1190–1192, 1985.

Massler, M.: Geriatric Dentistry: The Problem. *The Journal of Prosthetic Dentistry,* 2: 62–69, 1982.

McAuliffe, K. & McAuliffe, S.: Keeping Up with the Genetic Revolution. *The New York Times Magazine,* Nov. 6, 1983.

Motulsky, A.G.: Impact of Genetic Manipulation on Society and Medicine. *Science,* 219: 135–140, 1983.

Ortonne, J.P. & Thivolet, J.: Hair Melanin and Hair Color. *Hair Research.* Berlin: Springer-Verlag, 1981, pp. 146–162.

Ouslander, J.G.: Drug Therapy in the Elderly. *Annals of Internal Medicine,* 95: 711–722, 1981.

Ouslander, J.G. & Beck, J.C.: Defining the health problems of the elderly. *Annual Reviews of Public Health,* 3: 55–83, 1982.

Preston, T.A. & M.C.: Ageism Undermines Relations with Elderly. *Medical World News,* vol. 27, No. 2: 26, December 8, 1986.

Rebec, G.V. *et al:* Ascorbic Acid and the Behavioral Response to Haloperidol: Implications of the Action of Antipsychotic Drugs. *Science,* 227: 438–440, 1985.

Richelson, L.S. *et al:* Relative Contributions of Aging and Estrogen Deficiency to Postmenopausal Bone Loss. *New England Journal of Medicine,* 311: 1273–1275, 1984.

Riesenberg, D. & Breedlove, C. (Eds.): Contempo '86. *Journal of the American Medical Association,* 256: 2055–2126, 1986.

Rockstein, M. & Sussman, M.: *Biology of Aging*. Belmont, CA.: Wadsworth, 1979.

Rook, A. & Dawber, R.: *Diseases of the Hair and Scalp*. Boston: Blackwell, 1982.

Rosenfeld, A.: Stretching the Span. *Wilson Quarterly*, Vol. IX, No. 1, 96–106, 1985.

Rowe, J.W.: Clinical Research on Aging: Strategies and Directions. *New England Journal of Medicine*, 297: 1332–1336, 1977.

Rowe, J. W.: Health Care of the Elderly. *New England Journal of Medicine*, 312: 827–835, 1985.

Sacher, G.A. & Duffy, P.H.: Genetic Relation of Life Span to Metabolic Rate for Inbred Mouse Strains and Their Hybrids. *Federation Proceedings*, 38: 184–188, 1979.

Sady, P. *et al:* Prolonged Exercise Augments Plasma Triglyceride Clearance. *Journal of the American Medical Association*, 256: 2552–2555, 1986.

Schaumburg, H. *et al:* Sensory Neuropathy from Pyridoxine Abuse. *New England Journal of Medicine*, 309: 445–448, 1983.

Schneider, E.L. & Mitsui, Y.: The relationship between invitro cellular aging and in vivo human age. *Proceedings of the National Academy of Science, USA*, 73: 3584–3588, 1975.

Schneider, E.L. & Reed, J.D.: Life Extension. *New England Journal of Medicine*, 312: 1159–1168, 1985.

Siscovick, D.S. *et al:* The Incidence of Primary Cardiac Arrest During Vigorous Exercise. *New England Journal of Medicine,* 311: 874–877, 1984.

Smith, E.L., Reddon, W., & Smith, P.E.: Physical Activity and Calcium Modalities for Bone Mineral Increase in Aged Women. *Medical Science Sports Exercise,* 13: 60–64, 1981.

Smith, G.S., Walford, R.L., & Mickev, M.R.: Lifespan and Incidence of Cancer and Other Diseases in Selected Long-lived Inbred Mice and Their F1 Hybrids. *Journal National Cancer Institute,* 50: 1195–1213, 1973.

Snell, G.D.: Studies in Histocompatibility. *Science,* 213: 172–178, 1981.

Southgate, M.T. (Ed.): Contempo '84. *Journal of the American Medical Association,* 252: 2163–2354, 1984.

Stallones, R.A.: The Rise and Fall of Ischemic Heart Disease. *Scientific American,* 243: 53–59, 1980.

Summers, W.K. *et al:* Oral Tetrahydroaminoacridine in Long-Term Treatment of Senile Dementia, Alzheimer Type. *New England Journal of Medicine,* 315: 1241–1245, 1986.

Thorbecke, G.J. (Ed.): *Biology of Aging and Development.* New York: Plenum, 1975.

Timiras, P.S., Hudson, D.B. & Miller, C.: Developing and Aging Brain Serotonergic Systems. In *The Aging Brain: Cellular and Molecular Mechanisms of Aging in the Nervous System.* E. Giacobini *et al:* (Eds.) New York: Raven, 1982, pp. 173–184.

Walford, R.L.: *Maximum Life Span.* New York: Norton, 1983.

Williams, P.T. *et al:* Coffee Intake and Elevated Cholesterol and Apolipoprotein B Levels in Men. *Journal of the American Medical Association,* 253(10): 1407–1411, March 8, 1985.

Williams, T. *et al:* Impaired Growth Hormone Responses to Growth Hormone-Releasing Factor in Obesity: A Pituitary Defect Revised with Weight Reduction. *New England Journal of Medicine,* 311: 1403–1407, 1984.

Wood, W.G.: The Elderly Alcoholic: Some Diagnostic Problems and Considerations. In *The Clinical Psychology of Aging.* M. Storandt *et al.* (Eds.) New York: Plenum, 1978.

Wurtman, R.J.: Alzheimer's Disease. *Scientific American,* 252(1): 62–74, 1985.

Suggested Additional Reading

Berger, Stuart. *How to Be Your Own Nutritionist*. New York: Morrow, 1987.

Cousins, Norman. *Anatomy of an Illness As Perceived By the Patient*. New York: Norton, 1979.

DeVries, Herbert A. *Fitness After 50*. New York: Scribner's, 1987.

DuBos, Rene. *Celebrations of Life*. New York: McGraw-Hill, 1981.

Gould, Stephen Jay. *Ever Since Darwin: Reflections in Natural History*. New York: Norton, 1977.

Kevles, Daniel J. *In the Name of Eugenics: Genetics and the Uses of Human Heredity*. New York: Knopf, 1985.

Konner, Melvin. *The Tangled Wing: Biological Constraints on the Human Spirit*. New York: Holt, Rinehart and Winston, 1982.

Thomas, Lewis. *The Lives of a Cell*. New York: Viking, 1974.

Glossary

(Definitions, with a few exceptions, are from *Hammond Barnhart Dictionary of Science*, Robert K. Barnhart; Maplewood, N.J.: Hammond, Inc., 1986, and *Melloni's Illustrated Medical Dictionary*, Ida Cox, John Melloni, and Gilbert M. Eisner; Baltimore: The Williams and Wilkins Co., 1979. Both are excellent reference books.)

Actin—a protein found in muscle which acts in concert with another protein, myosin, to contract or expand the muscle.

Aerobic—respiration by using molecules of oxygen. Aerobic exercises such as dancing or jogging are possible because of rhythmic breathing, replenishing the flow of oxygen to the muscles.

Alveolar sacs—bags of air cells in the lungs.

Anaerobic—the metabolic process of tissue maintenance where there is a shortage of oxygen.

Amino acid conversion—a laboratory technique for measuring the number of cell duplications in living tissue, having value in determining age. Amino acids are organic compounds which group to form proteins.

Anecdotal—as used in medical and scientific writing, an explanation which lacks systematically-developed evidence; old wives' tales

Antigen—substance, such as toxins or bacteria, which stimulates the immune system to produce antibodies to counteract them.

Arteriosclerosis—hardening or stiffening of the arteries, a process which occurs in varying degrees in all of us during our lifetimes.

Atherosclerosis—a disease of the blood vessels, especially in arterial walls, manifested by lipid deposits which hasten the hardening of arteries and may even grow so large as to block blood flow.

Basal Ganglia—a group of structures at the base of the brain.

Beta-carotenes—particular crystalline pigments in carrots and other vegetable and fruit plants which the body converts to vitamin A.

Biomass technology—the use of plant matter or vegetation to produce fuel or energy.

Biotechnology—the manufacture of materials by use of molecular processes and properties. Synthetic insulin and monoclonal antibodies are products of biotechnology. The term also applies to techniques such as tissue-typing to identify genetic markers.

Catalase—an enzyme in the blood and tissues which assists or precipitates the hydrogen peroxide into water and oxygen.

Cerebellum—the portion of the brain, at the rear and base, which controls voluntary muscular movement.

Cerebrum—the large and rounded portion of the brain, composing the two cerebral hemispheres.

Cleavage enzyme—in genetics, a protein which "unzips" the two strands of the DNA molecule for RNA's transcription of hereditary information.

Chorionic Biopsy—tissue taken from the outer membrane enclosing the fetus. The term also denotes tests to determine sex and disease tendencies.

Chromosome—in the cell nucleus of plants and animals, a structure containing the DNA molecule which guards and transmits hereditary characteristics. Human cells normally have 46, or 23 pairs of chromosomes. The mother and father contribute one of each pair.

Control—in scientific or medical experiments, a standard of comparison for verifying results. For example, if you want to test the efficacy of a new drug-medicine given to people with a disease, you will need to compare their health, after the drug regimen, to the health of similar persons who did not take the drug. The latter group is called the "control."

Cytoplasm—the substance of a cell surrounding the nucleus, carrying structures within which most of the life processes of a cell take place.

Diastole—the rhythmic relaxation of the muscles of the heart chambers during which time they fill with blood. (see "Systole")

Diverticular disease—a condition marked by protrusions (diverticula) in the intestine; defects which impede the absorption of nutrients.

DNA (deoxyribonucleic acid)—the molecular basis of heredity present in chromosomes; it is responsible for the replication of proteins and nucleic acid.

Endocrine system—the body's glands which secrete hormones directly into the bloodstream. Also called ductless glands.

Endogenous—originating within the body.

Epithelium—a nonvascular, cellular layer that covers the internal and external surfaces of the body. Our skin is our external epithelium. The esophagus and most organs have epithelial surfaces.

Estrogen—a general term for the female sex hormones which are responsible for stimulating the development and maintenance of female secondary sex characteristics. Formed in the ovary, placenta, testis, adrenal cortex, and some plants. Therapeutic uses (with natural or synthetic preparations) include the relief of menopausal symptoms and amelioration of cancer of the prostate.

Estrus—in mammals, the cycle of changes in the genital tract produced by ovarian hormones.

Exogenous—originating outside the body. "Exogenous obesity" means that someone has gained weight because he eats too much food.

Fat mass—a term which signifies the abundance of fatty tissue in the body, as opposed to the "lean mass" of normally metabolizing, oxygenated tissue.

Free radical—a group of atoms with unshared electrons available for reaction. A "radical" is a group of atoms which can pass from one compound to another, forming a basic part of a molecule.

Genetic (biological) clock—an innate mechanism in organisms which controls the rhythm or cycle of various living functions such as photosynthesis in plants. In gerontology, a theory has it that the genetic clock contains the schedule for development, reproduction, and death.

Genetics—the science of heredity, especially the study of the origin of the characteristics of the individual and hereditary transmission.

Gerontology—the branch of scientific and medical study which investigates the changes of aging—physical and social—especially in elderly people.

Glomerulonephritis—kidney disease marked by alteration in the structure of the glomeruli (groups of tiny capillaries which provide filtration in the kidneys).

Glutathione—a substance in the blood which activates certain proteins and takes part in oxidation processes.

Hirsute—hairy. "Hirsutism" is excessively hairy.

Histamine—a white substance released in the body and which causes bronchiolar constriction, arterial expansion, increased gastric secretion, and a fall in blood pressure.

Homeostasis—a state of equilibrium in the physical and chemical functions maintained within an organism or an individual, such as temperature, blood pressure, and chemical content.

Hormonal axis—a cycle of interacting hormones, one of which stimulates the release of another, and so on, as in a chain reaction.

Immune complex—antigen-antibody clusters usually eliminated by the body but which sometimes linger, causing hypersensitive reactions.

In vitro—in an environment outside the body, usually a test tube or similar artificial environment.

In vivo—within the living body.

Involution—a retrograde process resulting in lessening in size of a tissue, as the return to normal size of the uterus after childbirth or the reduction of cellular mass of some organs during aging.

Isotonic—of equal tension or pressure, as between two muscles.

Leukocytes—white blood cells constituting a quarter to a third of all the white blood cells of the body and which respond to antigens either by directly destroying them or by triggering other types of immune defense.

Life expectancy—a statistically-devised measure of the age at which half of society's individuals die.

Life span—the actual years of life of an individual or a species.

Lipid—the fats and fat-like materials which, together with carbohydrates and proteins, constitute the main structural substance in the living cell.

Lipofuscin—a golden-brown, lipid-containing pigment which represents the indigestible portion of lysed material, associated with normal wear and tear; sometimes called the old age pigment.

Lymphocytes—white blood cells constituting a quarter to a third of all the white blood cells of the body and which respond to antigens either by directly destroying them or by triggering other types of immune defense.

Lyse—usually used as a suffix, for example, "hydrolysis," meaning the disintegration, dissolution, separation, or rupture of cells.

Metastasis—the transfer of a disease from its primary site to a distant location.

Mitochondria—compartmentalized structures present in the cytoplasm of almost all living cells which are responsible for generating usable energy by the formation of ATP. The average cell contains several hundred mitochondria.

Molecular biology—the branch of biology dealing with the

formation, structure, and activity of molecules essential to life, such as nucleic acid and protein molecules and their roles in cell replication and the transmission of genetic information.

Molecular genetics—the branch of genetics dealing with heredity and variation in the sequence of nucleotide bases of the genetic code.

Monoclonal antibody—an antibody produced in the laboratory by fusing genetically distinct cells and cloning the resulting hybrid so that each hybrid cell produces the same antibody.

Myelin—a fatty substance that forms a major component of the sheath that surrounds and insulates the axon of some nerve cells.

Myosin—the thick filaments of protein molecules in the muscles which react with actin to cause muscular movement.

Neurofibrillary tangle—a jumbled, disordered array of nerve fibrils, slender filaments which normally run parallel to the axon of the nerve.

Neuropathy—any disease of the nervous system affecting motor or sensory functions.

Nucleic acids—chemical compounds of the utmost biological importance, contained in all living organisms in the form of deoxyribonucleic acid (DNA) and ribonucleic acid (RNA).

Nucleotides—compounds into which nucleic acid splits when the elements of water are added, illustrating the sugar, nitrogen, and phosphate makeup.

Oligonucleotide—a compound made up of a small number of nucleotides (two to ten).

Pathogen—any microorganism or substance capable of causing disease.

Pathogenesis—the origin or development of a disease.

Peristalsis—the alternate contraction and relaxation of the walls of a tubular structure by means of which its contents are moved forward, characteristic of the intestinal tract and the esophagus.

Peroxidase—an enzyme found in plants and animals which facilitates oxidation by causing the decomposition of peroxides which liberate oxygen.

Phospholipids—a class of waxy or greasy compounds which contain phosphoric acid; most of them occur in tissues, especially membranes, such as the myelin sheath of nerve cells and red blood cell membranes.

Progeria—premature old age.

Protein—complex nitrogenous substances of high molecular weight that contain amino acids as their fundamental structural units, are present in the cells of all animals and plants, and function in all phases of chemical and physical activity of the cells.

Pyelonephritis—inflammation of the kidney; also called pyelitis.

Recombinant DNA—term describing the "technology" of formation of gene combinations that were not present in either parent.

Replication—the process of duplicating something, such as the repeated formation of the same molecule (as RNA "replicates" DNA).

Retinopathy—any degenerative non-inflammatory disease of the retina.

Ribosome—one of the tiny granules free in the cell's cytoplasm or attached to its endoplasm, containing a high concentration of RNA; it plays an important role in protein synthesis.

Soluble—capable of being dissolved.

Staphylococcus—a family of disease-causing bacteria.

Stem cells—a residual population of cells that retain the ability to divide.

Stochastic—a mathematical term having to do with random variables involving chance or probability. In gerontology, it has been applied to "wear and tear" or the variable events of life influencing an individual's rate of aging.

Subcutaneous—located beneath the skin; also called hypodermic.

Systemic—affecting the whole body.

Systole—the rhythmic contraction of the muscles of the heart chambers.

Thoracic—relating to the area of the chest.

Translation—the process in which the genetic data present in a messenger-RNA molecule direct the order of the specific amino acids during protein synthesis.

-trophic or -tropic—a suffix which means to turn toward or have an affinity for.

Viscosity—the resistance of a substance's capacity to flow due to molecular cohesion.

Index

ORDER FORM

10% DISCOUNT on orders of $20 or more —
20% DISCOUNT on orders of $50 or more —
30% DISCOUNT on orders of $250 or more —
On cost of books for fully prepaid orders

NAME

ADDRESS

CITY/STATE   ZIP

COUNTRY (outside USA)   POSTAL CODE

TITLE	QTY	PRICE	TOTAL
The New A-Z of Women's Health	|	@ $16.95	
Healthy Aging (paperback)	|	@ $11.95	
Healthy Aging (hard cover)	|	@ $17.95	
Lupus	|	@ $ 6.95	
Menopause Without Medicine	|	@ $11.95	
Nutirition and Your Body	|	@ $ 9.95	
Once A Month *4th Edition*	|	@ $ 9.95	
PMS: Premenstrual Syndrome *3rd Edition*	|	@ $ 7.95	
Sexual Healing	|	@ $12.95	

Shipping costs:
*First book: $2.00
($3.00 for Canada)
Each additional book:
$.50 ($1.00 for
Canada)
For UPS or First Class
rates and bulk orders
call us at (714)
624-2277*

TOTAL PRICE   _____
Less discount @_____%   (   )
TOTAL COST OF BOOKS   _____
Calif. residents add sales tax   _____
Shipping & handling   _____
TOTAL ENCLOSED
Please pay in U.S. funds only

❏ Check   ❏ Money Order   ❏ Visa   ❏ M/C

Card # _____ Exp date _____

Signature _____

Phone number _____

Complete and mail to:
Hunter House Inc., Publishers
PO Box 847, Claremont, CA 91711
❏ Check here to receive our book catalog